MW00718774

Lab Values for Nurses

Must Know Labs With Easy Memorization Tricks and Nursing Implications

Dr. Gabriel J. Connor

Table of Contents

INTRODUCTION

T o offer holistic care to patients, nurses and health care workers need to identify abnormal laboratory values and diagnostic data. Although the onus of diagnosis and ordering lab tests lies with the physician, it is important for nurses to be aware of the purpose of tests, their meaning, and the normal ranges for each one being ordered.

The ability to identify normal and abnormal values of a lab test is an important asset to make an informed clinical decision as a nurse. Laboratory tests are tools that give invaluable information and insight about a patient and help in care and honing nursing acumen. Lab tests aid in confirming the diagnosis, provide the prognosis of an illness, and suggest the patient's response to treatment.

The laboratory values are an important part of the NCLEX, yet some values give no indication of the normal range of lab levels. It is the responsibility of nursing personnel to identify whether lab values are within the normal range or not as it is of vital import. Note that laboratory values will vary from institution to institution.

Easy memorization tricks to help on exams are in a separate chapter of this book. You can glance through this single chapter just before the exams rather than sifting through all chapters if there is a time constraint.

BASIC PROCEDURES

A phlebotomist or certified nurse with training in blood specimen collection is allowed to perform venipuncture for the purpose of blood sample collection. The procedure includes the following steps:

- Identify the patient: ask his or her name and date of birth and explain the rationale and test procedure.
- Proper position: blood specimens are best drawn in a sitting position, and the patient should remain in the same position without movement for a minimum of 5 minutes before the sample is drawn.
- Confirm the lab test requested: look at the laboratory form for the ordered test, the patient information, and other requisites like allergies, fasting, dietary restrictions, and medications.
- Offer comfort: make sure the patient is not wearing tight clothing that could constrict the upper arm. The arm is to be placed in a gravitating position.
- Ensure proper hand hygiene: hands should be washed properly before wearing gloves.
- Identify the vein: inspect the patient's arm for an easily accessible vein for venipuncture, and then the tourniquet is to be applied 3 to 4 inches above the chosen site. Ensure that the tourniquet is not too tight and do not leave it on for more than 2 minutes.
- Prepare the site: cleanse the area of the chosen vein using alcohol in circular movements, beginning at the center of the site and working outward.
- Draw the sample: ask the patient to make a fist. Hold the patient's arm using your thumb firmly to make the skin taut and position the vein to prevent it from slipping at an angle of 15 to 30º. Gently insert the needle through the skin into the lumen of the vein.
- Fill the tube: collect the amount of blood sample required and then remove the tourniquet.

- Remove the needle: in a single and swift motion, remove the needle from the patient's vein and apply pressure with a folded gauze over the venipuncture site for 1 to 2 minutes.
- Label the tube: the tube should be labeled correctly with the patient's name, birth date, hospital identification number, time, and date of the sample collected.
- Transport specimen: the specimen should be delivered to the laboratory immediately for processing and analysis.

NOTES

_____
_____
_____
_____
_____
_____
_____
_____
_____
_____
_____
_____
_____
_____
_____
_____
_____

Diagnostic testing has three phases: pretest, intratest, and post-test. Each phase involves different roles and responsibilities.

PRETEST

In the pretest, the primary focus is on preparing the patient for the procedure. Responsibilities include:

- Assessment of the patient to determine precautions for the procedure
- Preparation of the equipment and supplies needed
- Preparation of a consent form, if required
- Providing information and answering queries of the patient about the procedure

INTRATEST

The intratest focuses mainly on specimen collection and performing or assisting with certain diagnostic procedures. Additional responsibilities during an intratest are:

- Standard precautions need to be employed, and sterile techniques to be used when indicated
- Monitoring the patient's response during the procedure and providing emotional support to the patient
- Ensure correct labeling, storage, and transportation of the specimen to the laboratory

POST-TEST

In the last part of diagnostic testing, nursing care is mainly focused on observations and patient follow-up. Additional responsibilities during post-test include:

- Comparison of previous and current test results
- The appropriate members of the healthcare team is to be notified of the results

ERYTHROCYTE STUDIES

A n erythrocyte called a red blood cell (RBC) is a type of cell produced in the bone marrow and found in the blood. Red blood cells develop in the fetal liver or the adult bone marrow via erythropoiesis. Erythropoiesis is a process stimulated by erythropoietin, a cytokine hormone, produced in the kidney when oxygen levels are low. RBCs are the primary cells in the body's respiratory system as they are responsible for carrying oxygen from the lungs to all the peripheral parts of the body via hemoglobin; and they are very important for nearly all the basic physiologic processes. The number of erythrocytes in the blood is usually part of a complete blood count (CBC) test.

The lab values related to red blood cell studies include hemoglobin, red blood cell count, hematocrit, erythrocyte sedimentation rate, and serum iron. Venous blood is used for an analysis of a complete blood count (CBC), a primary screening test ordered to give an idea of the health of a patient. Laboratories generally prefer venous blood since if there is any need to check or repeat a test, additional blood is already available without having to get another specimen from the patient.

Erythrocyte studies are used to look for conditions such as anemia, dehydration, malnutrition, and leukemia. Red blood cells are the most numerous cells of the body. In normal blood there are about 5 million red blood cells per microliter. The normal red blood cell or erythrocyte is shaped like a biconcave disc such that it is thicker at the periphery and thinner in the center. They undergo multiple tightly regulated processes in order to remodel their structure, starting with the loss of the complex organelles system and the consequent acquisition of the typical biconcave shape. The disc has rounded edges.

RBCs have a flexible structure, making them capable of deforming to travel through the smallest blood vessels - the capillaries. The RBC, especially due to its membrane, renders the aging RBC unfit to circulate, leading to its destruction by the liver, spleen, and reticuloendothelial system. The average RBC remains in circulation for about 120 days. The RBC has a thin semi-permeable covering membrane made up of lipids strengthened by proteins with attached carbohydrates. Red blood cells have a normal diameter of 7.3 micrometers. When stained, RBCs appear darker at the periphery and lighter in the center due to variations in hemoglobin in different parts of the cell.

The RBCs in the peripheral blood do not contain a nucleus. They lose their nuclei during maturation and just before their release from bone marrow where they are formed. However, certain disease conditions show nucleated RBCs in the peripheral blood. RBCs also have a tendency to collect together like a pile of coins, which is called the Rouleaux formation.

The most crucial function of the red blood cell is to carry oxygen from the lung to the tissues and bring back carbon dioxide from these tissues to the lungs for excretion. It also aids in maintaining an acid-base balance. As RBCs do not have nuclei and are no longer manufacturing proteins or other substances, they use very little oxygen for their own metabolism. Thus, they are very good oxygen carriers.

Red blood cells also induce vasodilation by mediating the effects of nitric oxide. They are involved in the process of thrombosis and hemostasis and have an important role in the immune response against pathogens.

NOTES

_____

_____

_____

_____

_____

_____

_____

_____

_____

RBCs or erythrocytes are biconcave-shaped cells that carry oxygen from the lungs to the tissues and carry carbon dioxide from the peripheral tissues to the lung. They have a lifespan of 120 days and are removed from the blood by the liver, spleen, and bone marrow, which are a part of the reticuloendo-thelial system.

NORMAL RANGES
- Male Adult: 4.5 - 6.2 million cells/cumm
- Female Adult: 4.5 - 5 million cells/cumm

INDICATIONS
To determine anemia, polycythemia, dehydration or response to treatment.

INTERPRETATION
RBCs increase either due to relative decrease in plasma as in hemoconcentra-tion or dehydration or as a result of an absolute increase in hematopoietin, as in renal cell carcinoma.

INCREASED LEVELS
Hemoconcentration, dehydration, smokers, acute stress, polycythemia vera, high altitude and renal cell carcinoma.

DECREASED LEVELS
Anemias, hemolysis, hemorrhage, failure of marrow production, chronic re-nal failure.

INTERFERING FACTORS
Conditions that increase plasma volume like pregnancy do not reflect abso-lute anemia. Conditions like dehydration do not reflect absolute polycythe-mia due to decreased plasma volume.

NURSING IMPLICATIONS
Explain the procedure of the test, encourage avoiding stress, and explain that fasting is not required. Apply a dressing over the puncture site, monitor the puncture site for oozing and hematoma formation. Then the patient can re-sume normal activities and diet.

Hemoglobin is a protein component of red blood cells that acts as a carrier for oxygen and carbon dioxide transport. It is composed of heme (a pigment) that carries iron, and globin (a protein).

NORMAL RANGES
- Male adult: 14 - 16.5 g/dl
- Female adult: 12 - 16 g/dl
- Critical values: <5 g/dl or >20g/dl

INDICATIONS
To measure severity of anemia or polycythemia and to monitor response to therapy.

INTERPRETATION
Low hemoglobin indicates anemia, characterized by an insufficient RBC count to deliver oxygen to peripheral tissues. High hemoglobin indicates polycythemia when the hemoglobin is more than 18.5g/dl in men and 16.5g/dl in women.

INCREASED LEVELS
Polycythemia vera, burns, chronic obstructive pulmonary disease, congenital heart disease, congestive heart disease, dehydration.

DECREASED LEVELS
Anemia, nutritional deficiency, hemolysis, hemorrhage, lymphoma, kidney disease, splenomegaly, cancer, neoplasia.

INTERFERING FACTORS
Conditions that cause changes in plasma volume without changes in overall RBC cell count can also affect the Hb and may lead to relative anemia or relative polycythemia.

NURSING IMPLICATIONS
Manage fatigue, maintain adequate nutrition, maintain adequate perfusion and encourage patient compliance with prescribed therapy.

Hematocrit is the volume of packed red cells in a particular specimen of blood calculated as a percentage of total volume of blood.

NORMAL RANGES
- Male adult: 42 -52%
- Female adult: 35 - 47%

INDICATIONS

Hematocrit shows that a patient has anemia, erythrocytosis, or changes in plasma volume. Hematocrit value is used as a cutoff to determine the amount of requirement for transfusion.

INTERPRETATION

Hematocrit is raised with an increase in the number of red blood cells or a decrease in plasma volume. Hematocrit falls in decreased erythropoiesis or hemolysis and hemorrhage where plasma volume is increased. Hematocrit may be measured by centrifugation or automated methods.

INCREASED LEVELS

Polycythemia vera, burns, COPD, congenital heart disease, dehydration, eclampsia.

DECREASED LEVELS

Anemia, hemoglobinopathy, bone marrow failure, hemorrhage, hemolytic reaction, normal pregnancy, multiple myeloma.

INTERFERING FACTORS

People living in high altitudes have a high HCT. Hemodilution of pregnancy causes decreased HCT. Lower HCT is seen in men and women over the age of 60. Severe dehydration causes a false increase in HCT.

NURSING IMPLICATIONS

Manage fatigue, avoid complications of anemia, maintain adequate nutrition, maintain adequate perfusion, and encourage compliance with prescribed therapy.

Red blood cell indices determine the characteristics of an RBC. RBC indices aid in diagnosis of anemias and liver diseases.

Mean corpuscular volume (MCV): Average size of the individual RBC

Mean corpuscular hemoglobin (MCH): Hgb amount in one cell

Mean corpuscular hemoglobin concentration (MCHC): proportion of each cell occupied by the Hgb

NORMAL RANGES

Mean corpuscular volume (MCV): Male: 78 – 100 µm3; Female: 78 – 102 µm3

Mean corpuscular hemoglobin (MCH): 25 – 35pg

Mean corpuscular hemoglobin concentration (MCHC): 31 – 37%

INDICATIONS

RBC counts and RBC indices are used to diagnose different types of anemias.

INTERPRETATION

RBC indices can help to identify the cause of anemia. The MCV is the most important value in the RBC indices that help in identifying the type of anemia.

INCREASED LEVELS

HIGH MCV: vitamin B12 deficiency, Folate deficiency, Chemotherapy

HIGH MCHC: hereditary spherocytosis, sickle cell disease

DECREASED LEVELS

LOW MCV: iron deficiency, thalassemia, lead poisoning, chronic diseases

LOW MCHC: thalassemia, iron deficiency, lead poisoning

INTERFERING FACTORS

Hyperglycemia, hyperlipidemia, hyperuremia.

NURSING IMPLICATIONS

Explain the test procedure, encourage avoiding stress, explain that this test does not require fasting, apply manual pressure and dressing over puncture site and watch for oozing or hematoma formation.

Iron is essential for blood formation and helps in the transport of oxygen in the lungs to the peripheral tissues and carbon dioxide from the tissues to the lungs.

NORMAL RANGES

Male adult: 65 – 175 mcg/dL

Female adult: 50 – 170 mcg/dL

INDICATIONS

Helps in diagnosing anemias and hemolytic disorders.

INTERPRETATION

Iron deficiency anemia develops when stores of iron in the body fall too low to support normal red blood cell (RBC) production. Hemochromatosis is diagnosed when elevated serum iron levels are present, usually an incidental finding on routine screening.

INCREASED LEVELS

Hemochromatosis, hemosiderosis, hemolytic anemia, iron poisoning, hepatic necrosis, hepatitis, lead toxicity.

DECREASED LEVELS

Iron deficiency anemia, chronic blood loss, chronic hematuria, chronic pathologic menstruation, neoplasia, late stages of pregnancy.

INTERFERING FACTORS

If iron deficiency anemia patients are on iron supplements before blood is drawn, normal or high concentrations of iron are noted.

NURSING IMPLICATIONS

A recent intake of a meal containing high iron content may affect the results. Drugs that cause decreased iron levels include colchicine, deferoxamine, adrenocorticotropic hormone, testosterone, and cholestyramine. Drugs that can cause increased iron levels include iron preparations, dextrans, ethanol, estrogens, methyldopa, and oral contraceptives.

Erythrocyte sedimentation rate (ESR) is a valutation of the rate at which erythrocytes settle in a blood sample within one hour.

NORMAL RANGE

0-30 mm/hour (value depends on age)

INDICATIONS

indicated in diagnosis of acute or chronic infections, inflammation, tissue necrosis and infarction.

INTERPRETATION

Increased ESR levels indicate a current ongoing infection, inflammation, tissue necrosis and infarction.

INCREASED LEVELS

Bacterial infection, inflammatory disease, malignant diseases, chronic renal failure, hyperfibrinogenemia, severe anemia.

DECREASED LEVELS

Polycythemia vera, sickle cell anemia, hypofibrinogenemia and spherocytosis.

INTERFERING FACTORS

Technical factors such as room temperature, time from specimen collection, vibration, inclination/orientation of the ESR tube can affect the results of the test.

NURSING IMPLICATIONS

Fasting is not required, fatty meals before tests may alter the plasma factors

NOTES

_____

_____

_____

_____

_____

_____

WHITE BLOOD CELL AND DIFFERENTIAL

The leukocytes or white blood cells are another of the formed elements of the blood. The WBC (white blood cell count) is a count of the number of white blood cells in a certain volume of blood. They are present in lesser numbers than the RBC in the blood. They account for 1 WBC for every 500 RBC's. White blood cells (leukocytes) are classified into myeloid (neutrophils/polymorphs, eosinophils, basophils, monocytes) and lymphoid (lymphocytes). The neutrophils, eosinophils, and basophils are also called granulocytes because their cytoplasm contains granules. Leucocytes are larger than RBCs as they all have a nucleus.

An automated hematology analyzer performs the test.

The total white blood cell count is an absolute number, and the subtypes of white blood cells are given as a differential WBC count, expressed as an absolute number or as a percentage. Microscopy is done to study the nuclei and other characteristics of the WBC. A blood smear is prepared and stained with Giemsa stain or Leishman stain for microscopy.

The protection of the body against foreign bodies, infections, and other substances is the job of the white blood cells. The differential count provides specific information on subtypes of WBCs:

Neutrophils are the foremost common form of WBC and are the first line of defense against pyogenic infections. They are actively motile and get attracted to places where an infection is going on or are drawn by various chemical stimuli in the body. With the help of antibodies, the neutrophil can ingest (phagocytose), kill, and digest harmful organisms that enter the body.

Lymphocytes play an enormous role in response to inflammation or infection. They are mononuclear cells and are motile. They are divided into two main types: The B lymphocyte and the T lymphocyte. The B lymphocyte is derived from bone marrow precursors and are stimulated by the attachment to their membranes of specific antigens and create antibodies. These cells transform into plasma cells, which create specific immunoglobulins. The T lymphocytes processed in the thymus are responsible for tissue immunity, which is seen when these lymphocytes kill cells infected with virus. They also play a role in tissue response to organ transplants and certain tumor cells. Lymphocytes are not phagocytic but play a very important role in immunity against various infections.

Monocytes are large mononuclear and phagocytic cells that act by killing and digesting the foreign organism (phagocytosis), and they respond to infection, inflammation, and foreign bodies). They also act as scavengers to remove inert matter, foreign bodies, dead cells, and other substances. The monocyte in the blood is an earlier stage of the phagocytic cell in tissue, called a macrophage. The monocytes not only present the processed antigen to the lymphocyte but they also produce a substance that activates the T lymphocytes to proliferate. They secrete the plasminogen activator factor and some of the components of complement. They are also the main source of pyrogen, which causes body temperature to rise (fever).

Eosinophils are motile; they localize to substances released by mast cells and sensitized lymphocytes. They are also phagocytic. They are often found attached to foreign agents such as adult worms and are increased in allergic reactions and parasitic infections.

Basophils are the chief carriers of histamine in the blood, the release of which is associated with hypersensitivity and allergic reactions. They respond to allergies, inflammation, and autoimmune diseases. They also carry and release heparin. Band forms are the first immature WBCs that are released into the blood.

The production of WBCs occurs in the bone marrow by hematopoiesis by the multipotential progenitor cells/hematopoietic stem cells. They are a crucial part of the immune system and play a vital role in the body's defense mechanism. The WBC count and differential count are used to assess the body's response to benign and malignant conditions such as acute and chronic infections, inflammatory conditions, allergic reactions, immunodeficiency states, leukemias, and lymphomas. It is also used for assessing prognosis, response to chemotherapy, growth factors, and immunosuppression.

A white blood cell (WBC) count lower than 4000 cells/cumm is called leuko-penia. A count of more than 11000 cells/cumm is known as leukocytosis.

WBC count is decreased in hematopoietic stem cell disorders that do disrupt the normal growth and maturation in the bone marrow, as seen in myelodys-plastic syndrome, leukemia or when the supply is depleted by treatments such as chemotherapy or radiation therapy.

WBC count is elevated, that is leukocytosis, and seen in response to infection, inflammatory disorders (referred to as reactive leukocytosis), stress or abnor-mal production as in leukemia.

The malignant proliferation of white blood cells also causes leukocytosis. These abnormal clones of white blood cells show malignant proliferation in the bone marrow and are classified as lymphoid and myeloid neoplasms, de-pending upon the sub-type of white cell proliferation. These malignancies are further divided by the type of differentiation of the individual cell types and are classified as chronic leukemias such as chronic myeloid leukemia, chronic lymphocytic leukemia and acute leukemia conditions like acute myeloid leu-kemia and acute lymphoblastic leukemia.

NOTES

_____

_____

_____

_____

_____

_____

_____

_____

_____

_____

White blood cells are the first line of defense against foreign bodies and other substances. The WBC count assesses the total amount of white blood cells in a cubic millimeter of blood. The differential count provides specific information about the WBC subtypes: neutrophils, lymphocytes, monocytes, eosinophils and basophils.

NORMAL RANGE

WBC Count: 4500-11000 cells per cumm.

Neutrophils 55-70%, Lymphocytes 20-40%, Monocytes 2-8%, Eosinophils 1-4%, Basophils 0-2%.

INDICATIONS

A crucial part of our immune system are white blood cells; they protect our bodies against infection and other foreign substances. The white blood cell count and differential shows the body's response to acute and chronic infections, inflammatory conditions, allergic reactions, immunodeficiency states, leukemias and lymphomas.

INTERPRETATION

A leucocyte count of less than 4000 cells/cumm is leucopenia. A leucocyte count of more than 11000 cells/cumm is leukocytosis.

INCREASED LEVELS

Leucocytosis: inflammation, Infection, Leukemic neoplasia, stress, trauma

Neutrophilic leucocytosis: Acute bacterial infections, myocardial infarction, burns, crush injuries.

Lymphocytosis: viral infections, pertussis Accompanies monocytosis,

Eosinophilia: Allergic disorders, drug reactions, Parasitic infections

Basophilia: Rare allergic reactions and acute leukemias

DECREASED LEVELS

Bone marrow failure, autoimmune disease, congenital aplasia, drug toxicity.

INTERFERING FACTORS

Acute physical or emotional stress can cause an elevated leukocyte count.

NURSING IMPLICATIONS

A "shift to the right" indicates that the neutrophils are mature and have more nuclear segments than usual. A "shift to the left" indicates more immature neutrophils in the blood.

COAGULATION STUDIES

In the normal adult, about 5 liters of liquid blood are being pumped around the body through the circulatory system. The body has mechanisms to keep all that blood in a fluid state as it circulates, while also having the potential to gel or coagulate should it become necessary. Other mechanisms maintain and repair any damage to the vessels, which result in leakage. Yet other and mechanisms reliquefy blood that has clotted in order to reopen vessels that become closed or occluded (thrombosed).

There is normally a constant and dynamic balance between the various forces or mechanisms involved in hemostasis. Hemostasis is a word used that includes all the factors and mechanisms that help keep the circulating blood fluid, maintain the integrity of the vessel wall, and control bleeding if a vessel break occurs. The term hemostasis thus includes coagulation of the plasma and the mechanisms and actions of the blood vessel themselves, along with the contribution of platelets.

Generally, one needs normal functioning of all three components (vessels, platelets and plasma) to ensure normal hemostasis. Usually, a mild dysfunction can be compensated by one or both of the others so there is no clinical problem, no bleeding. and no thrombosis - at least without major trauma. A person with mild dysfunction might never have had any bleeding over years of normal life only to develop major bleeding during surgery or after being in a major accident. On the other hand, if two or all three of the components have some abnormality at the same time, then clinical dysfunction is nearly always seen.

Coagulation studies are done to assess the clotting function in an individual. The panel of tests include platelet count, prothrombin time, international normalized ratio, activated partial thromboplastin time, bleeding time, and D-dimer.

The hemostatic system is composed of platelets, coagulation factors, and the endothelial cells lining the blood vessels. The fragmentation of the cytoplasm of megakaryocytes generates platelets in the bone marrow, and they circulate in blood as tiny anucleate disc-shaped particles with a lifespan of 7-10 days. Normally thrombosis is prevented by the endothelial cell linings' resistance to interacting with platelets and coagulation factors. When there is injury to the endothelial continuity, the underlying matrix gets exposed, and a continuous series of events are set in action to seal the primary defect (primary hemostasis). Platelets interact with the subendothelium-bound von Willebrand factor (vWf) via the membrane glycoprotein (GP) Ib complex and play a primary role in this process. This initial interaction (platelet adhesion) leads to other adhesive reactions that allow the platelets to aggregate and form a clot.

The coagulation pathway needs to be understood to interpret prothrombin time (PT). A measure of the integrity of the extrinsic and final common pathways of the coagulation cascade gives the prothrombin time. It is made up of tissue factor and factors VII, II (prothrombin), V, X, and fibrinogen. Thromboplastin, an activator of the extrinsic pathway and calcium, is added to the blood sample and then the time (in seconds) is noted that is required for fibrin clot formation.

Partial thromboplastin time (PTT) and activated partial thromboplastin time (aPTT) are used to test the same function, but in aPTT test, an activator is added to speed up the clotting time and therefore a narrower reference range is obtained. The aPTT is more sensitive than PTT and is therefore preferred to monitor the patient's response to heparin therapy.

The international normalized ratio is a standardized number and deduced in the lab; therefore, it varies from institute to institute. It is important to check INR in patients on anticoagulants, also called blood thinners or anti-clotting medicines. The INR is deduced using prothrombin time (PT) test results. INR measures the time taken for blood to clot and is an international standard for the PT. The INR test is done to see how well the blood clots.

Bleeding time is a test to assess the body's ability to form a clot as well as platelet function. The test involves pricking a needle in a superficial area of the skin and monitoring the duration of time needed for bleeding to stop (i.e., the bleeding site turns "glassy").

D-dimer is the degradation product of crosslinked (by factor XIII) fibrin. The current activation of the hemostatic system is identified by this test. The reference range of D-dimer is < 250 ng/mL, or < 0.4 mcg/mL.

Each laboratory establishes a reference range/cutoff value for D-dimer or, if a lab wants to use a published cut off value from the literature, the same methodology should be used to determine the value and preferably from the same manufacturer.

Latex agglutination–based kits are available for point-of-care testing to determine the semiquantitative amount of D-dimer. This test is less clinically valuable as it has high interobserver variability.

An automated point-of-care D-dimer test has been developed that gives quantitative results, providing an excellent, cost-effective, and rapid tool, especially in the emergency setting to rule out pulmonary embolism among patients with a low probability of occurrence.

NOTES

The production of platelets occurs in the bone marrow by the fragmentation of megakaryocytes and play a vital role in hemostasis. Platelets function in hemostasis, retraction of the clot, and activation of coagulation factors.

NORMAL RANGE
150,000 to 400,000 cells/mm^3

INDICATIONS
Platelets are counted to diagnose and monitor diseases and also to look for the causes of excessive bleeding or clotting.

INTERPRETATION
A platelet count of less than 150000 cells/cumm is thrombocytopenia and platelet count of more than 4,00000 cells/cumm is thrombocytosis.

INCREASED LEVELS
Iron deficiency anemia, post splenectomy, polycythemia vera, rheumatoid arthritis and malignant disorders.

DECREASED LEVELS
Immune thrombocytopenia, thrombotic thrombocytopenia, disseminated intra vascular coagulation, cancer, chemotherapy, hemorrhage, haemolytic anemia, and infection.

INTERFERING FACTORS
Platelet clumps are formed in capillary collections. Viral infections, drugs and chemotherapeutic medicines also cause platelet aggregates.

NURSING IMPLICATIONS
In thrombocytopenia, the venipuncture site should be assessed. Increased platelets are seen in high altitudes, persistent cold temperature, and strenuous exercise. Caution should be observed in patients with low platelet counts for bleeding.

APTT evaluates the length of time to form a blood clot. It is a measure of the intrinsic and coagulation pathway sequence. It gives the measurement of the amount of time required for citrated recalcified plasma to clot after partial thromboplastin is added to it. It is a screening test for deficiencies and inhibitors of all factors, except factors VII and XIII.

NORMAL RANGE:
20 to 60 seconds (depends on the activator used).

INDICATIONS
To monitor heparin therapy, detects coagulation disorders of hemophilia A and hemophilia B.

INTERPRETATION
A normal APTT with an abnormal PT means that the extrinsic pathway has a defect. An abnormal APTT with normal PT means that the intrinsic pathway is defective.

INCREASED LEVELS
Disseminated intravascular coagulation, hemophilia, heparin administration, Congenital clotting factor deficiency, leukaemia, a vitamin K deficiency.

DECREASED LEVELS
Disseminated intravascular coagulation in the early-stage of cancer.

INTERFERING FACTORS
Certain drugs prolong the values. Incorrect blood to citrate ratio may alter values. A high or low hematocrit alters values.

NURSING IMPLICATIONS
Samples should be drawn from an arm into which a heparin infusion is not being given. Apply manual pressure to the venipuncture site. The blood specimen should be transported to the laboratory immediately, The aPTT should measure between 1.5 and 2.5 times the normal if the patient is receiving heparin anticoagulation therapy. Signs of bleeding should be looked for if the aPTT value is more than 90 seconds.

Prothrombin is essential for fibrin clot formation; it is a vitamin K-dependent glycoprotein produced in the liver. The PT gives the measure of the amount of time taken in seconds for formation of the clot. The international normalized ratio (INR) is used to monitor the effectiveness of Warfarin and is deduced from the result of PT.

NORMAL RANGE

Normal: 11 – 13 seconds.

Critical value: >20 seconds for patients not on **anticoagulants**.

The INR is calculated in each laboratory and is specific to the thromboplastin reagent used. INR standardizes the PT.

INDICATIONS

Screen for extrinsic clotting system dysfunction screening, monitor response to Coumadin therapy.

INTERPRETATION

A prothrombin time (PT) test diagnoses excessive clotting and a bleeding disorder. The international normalized ratio (INR) is deduced from a PT result and is used to monitor the response of a blood-thinning medication.

INCREASED LEVELS

Disseminated intravascular coagulation, Coumarin ingestion, hereditary factor and vitamin K deficiency, bile duct obstruction, hepatitis.

DECREASED LEVELS

Blood clots rapidly due to supplements and food containing vitamin K.

INTERFERING FACTORS

Certain drugs may prolong the values. Incorrect blood to citrate ratio may alter values. Hematocrit results may alter values.

NURSING IMPLICATIONS

Do not draw samples from an arm where there is a heparin infusion. Apply pressure to the venipuncture site. The blood specimen should be transported to the laboratory immediately. Check for signs of bleeding if the aPTT value is more than 90 seconds.

Bleeding time is done to assess the hemostatic function.

NORMAL RANGE

Duke method: 1 to 3 minutes

Ivy method: 3 to 6 minutes

INDICATIONS

Useful in detecting disorders of platelet function.

INTERPRETATION

It helps in assessment of platelet response to injury and vasoconstrictive ability).

INCREASED LEVELS

Disseminated intravascular coagulation, Glanzmann's thrombasthenia, Henoch-Schonlein Syndrome, clotting factor deficiency, bone marrow failure, Bernard-Soulier Syndrome, severe liver disease, thrombocytopenia, Uremia, Von Willebrand's disease, capillary fragility, collagen vascular disease, connective tissue disorder, Cushing's Syndrome, hereditary telangiectasia, hypersplenism, leukemia.

INTERFERING FACTORS

Anything that alters platelet function can interfere with bleeding time. Examples include aspirin, thrombocytopenia, and uremia. The test procedure and subjective observation by the technician performing the test are also factors that can interfere with the results.

NURSING IMPLICATIONS

Assess and confirm that the patient has not been on anticoagulants, aspirin, or aspirin-containing products for 3 days prior to the test. Inform the patient about the procedure of the test. Apply pressure dressing to patients with bleeding tendencies after the procedure.

NOTES

_____

_____

_____

_____

_____

_____

_____

D-Dimer is a test done to measure formation and lysis of a clot that results from the fibrin degradation.

NORMAL RANGE:

< 500 ng/mL

INDICATIONS

Aids in diagnosis of the formation of thrombus, helps to diagnose disseminated intravascular coagulation, monitors the effectiveness of therapy.

INTERPRETATION

A low level of d-Dimer indicates no clotting disorder and high levels of d-Dimer indicates a probable clotting disorder.

INCREASED LEVELS

Deep vein thrombosis, blood clotting disorders, pulmonary embolism, pregnancy, recent surgery.

INTERFERING FACTORS

Pregnancy, cigarette smoking, trauma, infection, sepsis, elderly patients, immobilized patients, autoimmune diseases can cause elevation of d-Dimer levels.

NURSING IMPLICATIONS

Inform the patient regarding the test, disease, and treatment. Monitor anticoagulation therapy, comfort the patient, encourage exercise and movement, positioning of the body, maintaining adequate tissue perfusion and preventing complications.

NOTES

_____
_____
_____
_____
_____
_____
_____

SERUM ELECTROLYTES

E lectrolytes are minerals that play an essential role in the most important bodily functions. Serum electrolytes are screening tests in patients with electrolyte and acid-base imbalances. The commonly ordered serum electrolyte panels include serum potassium, serum sodium, serum chloride, and serum bicarbonate.

Electrolytes are elements that are ionized in solution and migrate in an electric field. They are called cations or anions, depending upon whether they migrate toward the cathode or the anode. The major cations found in body fluids are sodium, potassium, calcium and magnesium. The major anions found in the body fluids are chloride, bicarbonate, phosphate and sulfate.

There are a number of other substances in body fluid that are ionized and carry an electric charge in a solution, including some organic acid radicals such as lactate, amino acids, proteins and various other trace elements. In this chapter, we discuss sodium, potassium, chloride, calcium, magnesium and phosphorus.

Electrolytes are involved in all body processes. They are involved in maintaining normal osmotic pressure as well as water distribution throughout the body both within the cell and the extracellular fluid. They are a major part of many metabolic processes. Any imbalance in electrolytes will have widespread effects in the body.

Serum potassium is an electrolyte and mineral in the blood whose value can be assessed by blood tests. Potassium has a narrow normal range and is vital to the function of the heart muscle and nerve cells. Potassium is ingested in food and beverages and primarily excreted through urine. A small portion is excreted through the gastrointestinal tract. Deranged potassium levels are notorious in causing irregular heartbeats or arrhythmias.

Serum sodium is routinely measured in assessing acid-base and water balance, electrolyte changes, as well as in assessing kidney function. Approximately 95% of the osmotically active substances in the extracellular compartment fluid is made up of sodium. Sodium is regulated by hormonal influences and any excess is removed by the kidneys, which carefully regulate the extracellular sodium.

Serum chloride exists in the extracellular space and is a predominant anion. Cellular integrity is maintained by chloride and its effects on water balance and osmotic pressure, along with maintaining acid-base balance. Chloride also has a major role in cardiovascular pathophysiology and neuronal pharmacology.

Serum calcium is one of the most abundant elements in the adult body. Calcium constitutes approximately 2% of adult body weight, which accounts for over 1 kg of calcium. All the calcium is contained in the bones as calcium hydroxyapatite, except 1%. All the calcium of the blood is present in the plasma. About 40% of serum calcium is attached to proteins.

About 10% exists as inorganic and organic anions of bicarbonate, lactate, and citrate; the rest of 50% of the calcium in circulation is free, known as ionized calcium. Calcium ions are essential to the functioning of the nervous system; the contractility of heart and skeletal muscles are maintained by calcium ions. Calcium is also associated with blood clotting and mineralization of the bone. The parathyroid hormone (PTH) and 1,25-hydroxy vitamin D tightly regulate the calcium concentration in circulation.

Elemental phosphorus is not found in free form in the body and only present as part of organic and inorganic compounds. Like calcium, about 85% of phosphates are present primarily in an inorganic form (hydroxyapatite) in our skeletons. Around 15% is present as organic compounds in our soft tissue and circulation.

Laboratory tests give a measure of organically bound phosphorus. The most important intracellular cation in the body is magnesium. Magnesium has a major role in normal neuromuscular activity, along with extracellular calcium. Additionally, intracellular magnesium is an important cofactor for nucleic acids, various enzymes and transporters that are vital for replication, energy metabolism, and normal cellular function.

Potassium serves important functions in the body such as regulating acid-base equilibrium, cellular water balance, and transmitting electrical impulses in skeletal and cardiac muscles. It is the most abundant intracellular cation.

NORMAL RANGE

3.5 - 5 mEq/L

INDICATIONS

Assesses renal function, cardiac function, gastrointestinal function and indicates the need for IV replacement therapy.

INTERPRETATION

Hyperkalemia occurs when the potassium level is more than the upper limit of the normal range. Hyperkalemias are notorious to cause lethal arrhythmias and hence one of the most important serum electrolytes.

INCREASED LEVELS

Acidosis, dehydration, acute or chronic renal failure, aldosterone-inhibiting diuretics, hemolysis, hypoaldosteronism, excessive IV intake.

DECREASED LEVELS

Diuretics, hyperaldosteronism, gastrointestinal disorders such as nausea and vomiting, ascites, burns, Cushing's syndrome, cystic fibrosis.

INTERFERING FACTORS

Platelet clumps are commonly seen in capillary collections. Viral infections, drugs and chemotherapeutic medicines are also prone to cause platelet aggregates.

NURSING IMPLICATIONS

Make a note on the laboratory request form if the patient is on potassium supplements. Falsely elevated potassium levels may be seen in patients with elevated white blood cell and platelet counts.

Sodium is a major extracellular fluid action that maintains osmotic pressure and acid-base balance. It also mediates transmission of nerve impulses. Sodium ion absorption takes place in the small intestine and is excreted in the urine, depending upon dietary intake.

NORMAL RANGE
135-145 mEq/L

INDICATIONS
Monitor the effectiveness of drugs, especially diuretics, on serum sodium levels. Determine whole-body sodium stores, as sodium is a predominantly extracellular ion.

INTERPRETATION
Hypernatremia occurs when serum sodium levels are higher than the upper limit of the normal range. Hyponatremia occurs when the sodium levels are lower than the lower limit of normal range.

INCREASED LEVELS
Diabetes insipidus, excessive IV sodium administration, excessive dietary intake, Cushing's Syndrome, excessive sweating, extensive thermal burns, hyperaldosteronism, osmotic diuresis.

DECREASED LEVELS
Chronic renal insufficiency, deficient dietary intake, diarrhea, diuretic administration, pleural effusion, ascites, Addison's disease, congestive heart failure, syndrome of inappropriate ADH (SIADH) secretion, vomiting or nasogastric aspiration.

INTERFERING FACTORS
Fluid imbalance, acute illness, and diuretics.

NURSING IMPLICATIONS
Blood samples should not be drawn from an extremity in which an intravenous (IV) solution of sodium chloride is infusing as it increases the level, producing inaccurate results.

Chloride is a salt of hydrochloric acid and one of the most abundant body anions in extracellular fluid. It acts as a buffer during oxygen and carbon dioxide exchange in red blood cells (RBCs) and also counterbalances cations like sodium. Chloride also helps in digestion as a part of the hydrochloric acid and in maintaining osmotic pressure and water balance.

NORMAL RANGE

95 – 105 mEq/L

INDICATIONS

Serum chloride assesses the water balance and acid base status.

INTERPRETATION

Chloride is an extracellular fluid anion that mainly exists as sodium chloride or hydrochloric acid. Hyperchloremia means high levels of serum chloride above the upper limit of the normal range, and hypochloremia means low levels of serum chloride below the lower limit of the normal range.

INCREASED LEVELS

Dehydration, metabolic acidosis, renal tubular acidosis, respiratory alkalosis, eclampsia, excessive infusion of normal saline, anemia, Cushing's Syndrome, hyperparathyroidism, hyperventilation, kidney dysfunction.

DECREASED LEVELS

Diuretic therapy, vomiting, hypokalemia, metabolic alkalosis, respiratory alkalosis, salt-losing nephritis, Addison's disease, aldosteronism, burns, chronic respiratory acidosis, congestive heart failure, syndrome of inappropriate antidiuretic hormone (siadh).

INTERFERING FACTORS

Excessive IV saline infusions can result in high values. Infants tend to have higher levels of chloride than adults and children. Certain drugs can alter chloride levels (i.e., loop diuretics, thiazide diuretics)

NURSING IMPLICATIONS

Any condition associated with prolonged vomiting, diarrhea, or both will alter chloride levels.

Sodium bicarbonate regulates the pH of body fluids and forms a part bicarbonate-carbonic acid buffering system of the body.

NORMAL RANGE:
22 to 29 mEq/L

INDICATIONS
Helps to diagnose an electrolyte imbalance, acidosis or alkalosis. Bicarbonate is part of a metabolic and electrolyte panel.

INTERPRETATION
It raises blood pH acts as a buffer against acidosis. Bicarbonate reacts with H+ ions to form water and carbon dioxide.

ACIDOSIS AND ALKALOSIS
Conditions or diseases that affect the lungs, kidneys, metabolism, or breathing is a potential to cause acidosis or alkalosis.

INTERFERING FACTORS
Metabolic alkalosis is a situation that increases the pH in tissues that causes a high level of bicarbonate in the blood. Metabolic alkalosis can be due to a loss of acid from the body, as seen during vomiting and dehydration.

NURSING IMPLICATIONS
Acidic or alkaline solutions ingestion may cause increased or decreased results.

Calcium (Ca+) is a cation that facilitates nerve impulse transmission, contraction of myocardial and skeletal muscles, and bone formation. Calcium is absorbed from dietary sources into the bloodstream and helps clotting of blood by converting prothrombin to thrombin.

NORMAL RANGE

Calcium (total calcium): 4.5 – 5.5 mEq/L (8.5 to 10.5 mg/dL)

Calcium (ionized): 2.5 mEq/L (4.0 – 5.0 mg/dL)

INDICATIONS

Serum calcium levels above 11.5 mg/dL cause symptoms. 12 mg/dL and above are critical values, and levels above 15 mg/dL is a medical emergency.

INTERPRETATION

Hypocalcemia is total serum calcium concentrations below the lower limit of the age and sex appropriate reference interval. Hypercalcemia occurs when the calcium levels are above the upper limit of the reference range.

INCREASED LEVELS

Hyperparathyroidism, hyperthyroidism, Paget's disease of the bone, acromegaly, granulomatous infections, lymphoma, metastatic tumor to the bone, renal or lung carcinoma.

DECREASED LEVELS

Hypoparathyroidism, Rickets, vitamin D deficiency, malabsorption, osteomalacia, pancreatitis, alkalosis, fat embolism, renal failure.

INTERFERING FACTORS

Drugs and bilirubin commonly compete with calcium for albumin binding.

NURSING IMPLICATIONS

Inform the patient that fasting may be required for 8 hours before the test. The patient should eat a normal calcium level diet for 3 days before the exam.

Phosphorus is present as phosphate and plays an important role in formation of the bone, buffering of acid-base, carbohydrate metabolism, and energy storage and release. Storage forms of high concentration of phosphorus are seen in the bones. Phosphorus is absorbed in the diet and excreted by the kidneys.

NORMAL RANGE
1.8 – 2.6 mEq/L (2.7 to 4.5 mg/dL)

INDICATIONS
Phosphate level measurement is useful in diagnosing and management of bone, renal disease, parathyroid disorders and a variety of other disorders.

INTERPRETATION
Serum phosphate levels of 1.5-2.4 mg/dL shows a moderate decrease.
Serum phosphate levels lower than 1.5 mg/dL cause red cell hemolysis, muscle weakness, impaired bone growth, and bone deformity.
Serum phosphate levels lower than 1 mg/dL are defined as critical and may be life-threatening

INCREASED LEVELS
Hypocalcemia, rhabdomyolysis, bone metastasis, renal failure, hemolytic anemia, hypoparathyroidism, sarcoidosis, acidosis, acromegaly, advanced myeloma or lymphoma, liver disease.

DECREASED LEVELS
Hypercalcemia, hyperparathyroidism, adult osteomalacia, childhood rickets, alkalosis, chronic alcoholism, diabetic acidosis, sepsis and malnutrition.

INTERFERING FACTORS
Specific drugs may interfere with the test results of serum phosphorous levels.

NURSING IMPLICATIONS
The patient should be informed that fasting may be required for at least 8-12 hours before the test.

Magnesium is used to determine the metabolic activity of the body and renal function. Magnesium is essential for the mechanism of blood clotting. It regulates neuromuscular activity and also plays the role of a cofactor for many enzymatic reactions. It is involved in calcium metabolism.

NORMAL RANGE
1.6 to 2.6 mg/dL

INDICATIONS
Patients with renal failure or gastrointestinal disorders need to be closely monitored and diagnosed for hypermagnesia or hypomagnesia. Patients with pre-eclampsia on magnesium sulfate need to be monitored.

INTERPRETATION
Serum magnesium levels of 1.0 mg/dL or lower manifest symptoms.
Serum magnesium levels of 9.0 mg/dL or higher may be critical and life-threatening.

INCREASED LEVELS
Renal insufficiency, hypothyroidism, ingestion of magnesium-containing antacids or salt, Addison's disease, uncontrolled diabetes.

DECREASED LEVELS
Chronic renal disease, hypoparathyroidism, malnutrition, chronic alcoholism, diabetic acidosis, malabsorption.

INTERFERING FACTORS
Phytate, fatty acids, and increased phosphate cause impairment in the absorption of magnesium. Hemolysis causes increased serum magnesium results because the RBC contains 2-3 times higher amount of magnesium than the serum.

NURSING IMPLICATIONS
Long-term parenteral nutrition therapy and prolonged use of magnesium supplements cause increased serum magnesium levels. Decreased serum magnesium levels are seen in an excessive loss of body fluids.

RENAL FUNCTION STUDIES

R enal function studies assess the kidney function of an individual. The chief functions of the organ are to regulate the water content and balance of the body, regulate electrolyte content, regulate the normal acid base equilibrium, retain various essential substances vital to the body, and excrete the waste products of metabolism, especially the end products of metabolism, urea and creatinine. The kidney excretes various organic acids as well as any increased inorganic substances in the diet and certain foreign substances.

Thus, the kidney has both a regulatory and excretory function. In addition, the kidney has an endocrine function since several hormones, including renin, help maintain arterial blood pressure and vascular tone. Erythropoietin which stimulates erythroid cell proliferation and maturation in bone marrow is secreted into the bloodstream by the kidney. The kidney is also a site of action of other hormones secreted elsewhere in the body, including the anti-diuretic hormone secreted by the posterior pituitary gland.

Also, both insulin and glucagon from the pancreas and aldosterone from the adrenal cortex are degraded in the kidney such that a conversion of vitamin D into its active form occurs, causing the retention of calcium by the renal tubules and the absorption of both calcium and phosphorus from the intestine. Thus, the kidney participates in bone metabolism.

The primary functional unit of the kidney is the nephron, which includes the glomerulus through which plasma is filtered. The various tests of renal function are classified either according to the regulatory, excretory or endocrine function or whether they measure glomerular filtration, tubular absorption, or tubular secretion.

Acute emergency to chronic settings can be assessed by renal function tests. These tests are primarily done to diagnose acute renal diseases to provide timely and appropriate treatment to the patient. Furthermore, renal function tests identify the stage or type of renal disease and also help in monitoring its prognosis. It is an important guide to assess the response to intervention.

Creatinine is the most essential value in a renal function test. It is an important marker of the glomerular filtration rate in blood. Its value in urine can be used as a quality control tool to assess the accuracy of a 24-hour collection. It may even remove the need for a 24 hour collection. Creatinine is formed constantly in the muscles at a steady rate. It is a dehydration product of creatine that cannot be reversed to creatine once formed. Therefore, the amount of creatinine varies with ethnicity, age, and gender as it is related to muscle mass and is formed on a daily basis.

Creatinine is not reabsorbed or secreted by the renal tubules once it is freely filtered through the glomerulus. The serum concentration of creatinine shows a balance between production and glomerular filtration rate (GFR). The creatinine clearance rate is an excellent surrogate for the glomerular filtration rate, particularly in patients whose muscle mass remains the same and GFR is constant.

The blood urea nitrogen (BUN) test is routinely obtained as part of a metabolic panel (basic or comprehensive). It plays an indispensable role in the emergency states as it gives valuable information about different types of clinical presentations.

In humans, urea and carbon dioxide are end products of the urea cycle and serve as alternative sources of energy. The amino acids present in food but not used in protein synthesis are oxidized and form urea and carbon dioxide.

About 85% of urea is excreted via the kidneys, and the remaining small portion is excreted via the gastrointestinal (GI) tract. In acute and chronic renal failure/impairment, serum urea levels increase as renal clearance is decreased in these conditions. Upper GI bleeding, dehydration, catabolic states, and high protein diets not related to renal conditions can also cause increased urea levels. Starvation and severe liver disease show decreased urea levels. When the BUN is increased, the ratio of BUN to creatinine can be useful to differentiate pre-renal from renal causes.

Serum creatinine is the most important indicator of renal function. Increased levels of creatinine reflect as a slowing of the glomerular filtration rate.

NORMAL RANGE
0.6 to 1.3 mg/dL

INDICATIONS
Creatinine value is vital in assessing renal function because it is an accurate reflection of the GFR. It is a marker of glomerular filtration rate in the blood and in urine and can be used as a tool of quality assurance to assess the precision of a 24-hour urine sample collection.

INTERPRETATION
Low serum creatinine values almost always reflect low muscle mass. Serum creatinine increases in acute kidney injury or chronic kidney disease where there is a decrease in GFR.

INCREASED LEVELS
Glomerulonephritis, nephritis, pyelonephritis, acute tubular necrosis, acromegaly, diabetic nephropathy, rhabdomyolysis, shock, urinary tract obstruction, congestive heart failure, dehydration.

DECREASED LEVELS
Muscular dystrophy, debilitation, myasthenia gravis.

INTERFERING FACTORS
Improper blood sampling may interfere with the results. Drugs interfering in creatinine estimation are ethamsylate, calcium dobesilate, and 5-aminolevulinic acid.

NURSING IMPLICATIONS
Patients should avoid excessive and strenuous exercise for 8 hours. Excessive intake of red meat for 24 hours before the test should be avoided.

Blood urea nitrogen is a substance formed by an enzymatic breakdown process of protein and formed in the liver. Urea goes through a free filtration in the renal glomeruli, with a small amount reabsorbed in the tubules and the remaining amount is excreted in the urine. Slowing of the glomerular filtration rate leads to elevation of Blood urea nitrogen.

NORMAL RANGE
8 to 25 mg/dL

INDICATIONS
BUN testing is asked as a part of a routine test panel. In an emergency setting it gives valuable information that helps to assess and diagnose various clinical presentations.

INTERPRETATION
If the blood urea nitrogen is elevated it indicates a slowing of glomerular filtration rate (GFR). The critical value of urea is >100 mg/dL and indicates serious renal function impairment.

INCREASED LEVELS
Glomerulonephritis, renal failure, nephrotoxic drugs, pyelonephritis, sepsis, ureteral obstruction, hypovolemia, myocardial infarction, shock, starvation, burns and congestive heart failure.

DECREASED LEVELS
Syndrome of inappropriate antidiuretic hormone (SIADH) or fluid overload, nephrotic syndrome, pregnancy, malnutrition.

INTERFERING FACTORS
A high-protein diet may cause high BUN levels. Medications like steroids and antibiotics can alter the values. A Low-protein diet may cause low BUN levels.

NURSING IMPLICATIONS
Red meat intake in excess should be avoided for 24 hours before the test, and strenuous exercise should be avoided.

GLUCOSE STUDIES

B lood glucose lab values are the most essential in managing diabetes mellitus. Blood sugar level is determined by the balance between absorption, storage and utilization. The body generally keeps the level of blood sugar amazingly constant despite periods of high absorption, that is, after meals and high utilization like exercise, fever, etc. There will be some variation, but the body keeps it within a certain normal range. When food is eaten and the level rises, more glycogen is made to store the excess sugar. Between meals and during exercise, glycogen is degraded to keep up blood sugar as glucose disappears from the blood for use in the tissues.

In diabetes mellitus, there is an upset in the balance of factors controlling the utilization of glucose. In most of the cases, the cause is a lack of sufficient insulin. Even in early and mild cases, where the fasting blood glucose is at the upper level of normal or only very slightly elevated, the rise in blood glucose after a meal is much more than normal, and it takes a long time for the elevated blood glucose to return to normal levels.

When the level of blood glucose exceeds 180 mg/dl, the amount filtered into the glomerular filtrate cannot all be reabsorbed, so the glucose appears in the urine (glycosuria). The level of blood beneath where no glucose appears in the urine is called the renal threshold. Normally this threshold is 180 mg/dl to 200 mg/dl. Renal glycosuria is a condition where the kidney has an unusually low threshold for glucose, and glucose appears in the urine even when the blood glucose is normal.

Glucose is a primary metabolite for energy production in the body. It is a monosaccharide. The digestive system breaks up the complex carbohydrates into the final product of monosaccharides like glucose, fructose or galactose. These broken down monosaccharides are then absorbed in the small intestine. The transport of glucose requires a specific transport protein and a simultaneous uptake of sodium ions into the cells. Glucose is closely regulated by hormones such as insulin, cortisol, and glucagon in blood circulation. These hormones regulate glucose entry into cells and impact various metabolic processes such as glycolysis, gluconeogenesis, and glycogenolysis. Glucose entry into the cells is mediated by glucose transporter (GLUT) receptors, a facilitated transport. GLUT-4 receptors are present in muscle and adipose tissues and require insulin for glucose transport, indicating their tissue specificity. Glucose is carried across the blood-brain barrier by a GLUT-1 receptor.

Glycolysis is the main metabolic reaction, using glucose as its substrate. Glycolysis is used by all tissues for the breakdown of glucose and to generate adenosine triphosphate (ATP), which is the principal energy producing molecule. It also serves as an intermediate for other metabolic pathways. Glycolysis serves as the core of carbohydrate metabolism.

Glucose tolerance testing (GTT) is indicated when a random or fasting blood glucose test is insufficient to diagnose or rule out diabetes mellitus. GTT is used to assess the ability of the body to regulate glucose metabolism. A combination of carbohydrate uptake from the gastrointestinal tract, peripheral glucose uptake, and hepatic glucose output is indicated by glucose tolerance test.

The GTT is done on an empty stomach in the morning, and the patient should remain seated throughout. This test measures the body's ability to handle a sudden large dose of glucose, determining both the effect on blood glucose and whether any glucose appears in the urine. The first sample is fasting glucose testing, after which the glucose load is administered orally or intravenously and plasma glucose is measured at specified intervals thereafter. In standard oral GTT, plasma glucose levels are measured at 2 hours after a 75 g oral glucose load, but for gestational diabetes mellitus, an additional sample may be measured at 1 hour. The recommended glucose is a maximum of 75 g, and the dosage for a child is 1.75 g/kg body weight.

A specific fraction of hemoglobin called hemoglobin A1c is found in patients with diabetes mellitus as well as healthy individuals. It is formed when the valine of N-terminal of the beta chain of hemoglobin A is modified by the addition of a component of sugar moiety. Hemoglobin A1c is stable once formed. Hence, the hemoglobin A1c level shows the average blood glucose for 120 days, which is the lifespan of a RBC.

It has been studied and shown that maintaining near normal levels of blood glucose as reflected by HbA1c delays the onset and also slows the progression of diabetic microvascular complications like retinopathy, nephropathy, and neuropathy. Even though finger prick measurement of glucose by patients remains the method of diabetes management and for adjusting daily insulin, the importance of ongoing, periodic A1c measurements to monitor compliance and the efficacy of therapy cannot be undermined.

NOTES

_____

_____

_____

_____

_____

_____

_____

_____

_____

_____

_____

_____

_____

_____

_____

_____

_____

Fasting blood glucose or sugar (FBS) levels are primary tests used to diagnose diabetes mellitus and hypoglycemia. Glucose is the essential source of cellular energy for the body and is essential for brain and RBC function.

NORMAL RANGE

Glucose, fasting: 70 – 110 mg/dL; Glucose, 2-hr postprandial: < 140mg/dL

INDICATIONS

Blood glucose levels are tightly regulated in a narrow range by a complex mechanism by several hormones. Hence, a derangement of variation of blood glucose is often a hint of illness.

INTERPRETATION

Values for diabetes mellitus:

- Fasting plasma glucose value of greater than 125 mg/dL
- Random plasma glucose more than 200 mg/dL, postprandial glucose at 2 hours >200 mg/dL
- Hypoglycemia is a blood glucose level < 70 mg/dL.

INCREASED LEVELS

Diabetes mellitus, corticosteroid therapy, Cushing's Syndrome, diuretic therapy, glucagonoma, pheochromocytoma, acute stress response.

DECREASED LEVELS

Insulinoma, extensive liver disease, hypopituitarism, hypothyroidism, insulin overdose, starvation.

INTERFERING FACTORS

Increased coagulation factor levels, the body's ability to produce and respond to insulin.

NURSING IMPLICATIONS

Fasting state of the patient for 8 to 12 hours is required before the test. The patients should withhold morning insulin or oral hypoglycemic medication if they are diabetic until the blood is drawn.

The glucose tolerance test (GTT) helps in the diagnosing diabetes mellitus. After injection or ingestion of glucose, If the glucose levels peak at higher than normal at 1 and 2 hours after and are slower than normal to return to fasting levels, a diagnosis of diabetes mellitus is confirmed.

NORMAL LAB VALUES FOR GTT
70 – 110 mg/dL (baseline fasting)
110 – 170 mg/dL (30 minute fasting)
120 – 170 mg/dL (60 minute fasting)
100 – 140 mg/dL (90 minute fasting)
70 – 120 mg/dL (120 minute fasting)

INDICATIONS
Oral GTT is indicated when the fasting or random blood glucose levels are suggestive toward the diagnosis of type 2 diabetes mellitus, for screening of impaired glucose tolerance, and to screen for gestational diabetes.

INTERPRETATION
Patients who present with a higher risk of developing diabetes mellitus, with a view to beginning preventive therapy, need a glucose tolerance test.

ABNORMAL GLUCOSE TOLERANCE TEST
Diabetes mellitus, glucagonoma, pheochromocytoma, corticosteroid therapy, Cushing's Syndrome, diuretic therapy, acute stress response.

INTERFERING FACTORS
Increased coagulation factor levels interfere with the glucose tolerance test results.

NURSING IMPLICATIONS
The patient should eat a carbohydrate-rich diet for 3 days before the test. Inform the patient to fast for 10 to 16 hours before the test. Patients with diabetes mellitus should withhold insulin or hypoglycemic medications. The patient should be informed that the procedure of the test may take 3 to 5 hours, require administration of glucose, oral or IV, and collecting of multiple blood samples.

HbA1c gives the measure of the amount of glucose attached to the hemoglobin. Hemoglobin is a part of the RBC that carries oxygen from the lungs to the peripheral organs. As the average lifespan of the RBC is about 3 months, the HbA1c gives a measure of the glucose levels over the past three months.

RESULTS

Normal range: less than 5.7%

Pre-diabetes: between 5.7%-6.5%

Diabetes : more than 6.5%

INDICATIONS

Diabetic symptoms: increased thirst, increased hunger, increased urination, fatigue, blurred vision. Higher risk of diabetes: severe hypertension, diabetes, obesity, sedentary lifestyle.

INTERPRETATION

HbA1c in the range of 4% to 5.6% indicates no diabetes.

HbA1c of 5.7% to 6.5% indicates a higher risk for diabetes mellitus.

HbA1c of greater than 6.5% indicates a diagnosis of diabetes mellitus.

INCREASED LEVELS

Uncontrolled diabetes mellitus, stress, Cushing's Syndrome, corticosteroid therapy, pheochromocytoma.

DECREASED LEVELS

Chronic renal failure Chronic blood loss, hemolytic anemia.

INTERFERING FACTORS

Anemia, disorders of the blood, high cholesterol levels, kidney diseases.

NURSING IMPLICATIONS

Early detection, screening and prevention of type 2 diabetes mellitus. Promoting self-care, promoting mental health, nutrition, urine monitoring, blood glucose monitoring, oral therapies, injectable therapies.

The diabetes mellitus autoantibody panel is used to detect type 1 diabetes and insulin resistance. It also identifies an insulin allergy in patients.

NORMAL VALUE FOR DM AUTOANTIBODY PANEL

<1:4 titer and no antibody should be detected

INCREASED LEVELS

Insulin resistance

Type I diabetes mellitus/ Insulin-dependent diabetes mellitus

Insulin allergy

Factitious hypoglycemia

NOTES

_____

_____

_____

_____

_____

_____

_____

_____

_____

_____

_____

_____

_____

_____

_____

ARTERIAL BLOOD GAS ANALYSIS

T he branching of the systemic arteries is like a tree in which the common trunk is the aorta that starts in the left ventricle while the smallest branches are capillaries that extend into the peripheral tissues of the body organs. Oxygenated blood is carried away from the heart to the peripheral tissues by large blood vessels called arteries.

Metabolism is the consumption of nutrients and release of acid metabolites. The accumulation of these acid metabolites should be prevented because major functions of the body like myocardial contractility and nervous system electrophysiology depend on an environment where a narrow range of free hydrogen ion concentration is present. The degree of free hydrogen ion concentration is the pH. If the normal ranges of pH deviate significantly and occur over short intervals, it could be life threatening. Thus, maintenance of the biologic system requires an exact acid base balance.

Almost 98% of metabolites are in the form of carbon dioxide. Carbon dioxide readily reacts with water to form carbonic acid, a substance that can reversibly exist in either a liquid or gaseous state. Since carbonic acid can be readily transformed into carbon dioxide, excretion of the normal metabolites can be achieved by the lungs (respiratory acid - base balance).

The normal gastrointestinal absorptive process provides nutrients whose metabolism results in approximately 1% to 2% of the acid load being organic and inorganic nonvolatile acids. All pathological metabolites are nonvolatile acids, and they cannot be excreted by the lungs. The mechanisms that provide for the buffering and accretion of nonvolatile acid metabolites is called metabolic acid base balance.

An arterial blood gas (ABG) sampling is done by direct puncture in the artery and is a procedure often practiced in the hospital emergency room and wards. Arterial blood sampling involves the violation of a blood vessel and hence caution should be exercised in three significant areas: bleeding, vessel obstruction and infection. Blood gas analysis uses an arterial sample cause only the left and right ventricles contain completely mixed blood returned from the capillary beds, where respiration has occurred.

Arteries are vessels in which virtually no gas exchange occurs; hence, the arterial sample is assumed to have the same pH, Po2 and Pco2 as the ventricle. The criteria to choose the site for an arterial sample should be based on safety, accessibility and patient comfort. The best site is the radial artery on the wrist because it is superficial in location, easy to palpate and stabilize, collateral circulation via the ulnar artery is excellent, the probing needle can be relatively pain free if the surrounding periosteum is avoided, and the artery is not adjacent to any major vein.

When the radial artery is the dominant blood supply to the palmar arch, the ulnar artery may be chosen as the puncture site. The ulnar artery is not the wrist artery of choice as it is difficult to stabilize and is more readily subjected to thrombosis, given its smaller diameter. The brachial artery in the antecubital fossa is an alternative choice when radial arteries are unavailable. It does have a few risks and, therefore, it is best done by the physicians. Non-physicians should be limited to radial arteries. Percutaneous cannulation of the dorsalis pedis artery is reliable, easily performed, and relatively safe. The femoral artery has been used in intensive care units for a long time without significant problems. If there is ischemia of the foot, it is an indication to remove the catheter immediately.

The ease of doing the procedure at the patient's bedside, the low incidence of major complications, and its rapid diagnostic yield make it an invaluable test to decide patient treatment by the medical personnel. It has very high value, especially in critically ill patients, to determine the exchange of gas in the blood.

ABG gives a lot of information on the acid-base balance in seriously ill patients. The determination of ventilation success is provided by the measure of CO2 content in ABG. Accurate determination of the alveolar-arterial oxygen gradient (A-a gradient) is only possible by ABG.

ABG results are indicative of the patient's condition at a specific point in time, and the clinical correlation should be done carefully as the clinical scenario progresses over time. The arterial blood gas test is indicated in assessment of respiratory, metabolic, and mixed acid-base disorders, which may or may not have physiologic compensation. In patients with diabetic ketoacidosis (DKA) on insulin infusion, ABG helps in monitoring the acid base status. ABG and venous blood gas (VBG) could be obtained simultaneously for comparison.

Response to therapeutic interventions can be monitored in patients on mechanical ventilation in respiratory failure. ABG aids in the assessment of the requirement for home oxygen therapy in patients with advanced chronic pulmonary disease. It also helps in the quantification of oxyhemoglobin and the quantification of the levels of carboxyhemoglobin and methemoglobin.

An ABG sampling is absolutely contraindicated if there is a local infection at the sample drawing site or distorted anatomy from congenital or acquired malformations, surgical interventions, or burns. Arteriovenous fistulas and severe peripheral vascular disease of the limb involved are also contraindications for the same. Severe coagulopathy, therapy with Warfarin, heparin and other anticoagulants, and the use of thrombolytic agents are relative contraindications.

NOTES

_____

_____

_____

_____

_____

_____

Arterial blood gases (ABGs) measure the extent of compensation by the buffer system. It gives a measure of pH and the levels of oxygen and carbon dioxide in arterial blood. Blood sampling is usually done from the veins, except for an ABG test where the blood is taken from an artery.

NORMAL VALUES

pH: 7.35 – 7.45, PaO2: 80 – 100 mmHg, SaO2: >95, PCO2: 35 – 45 mmHg, HCO3: 22 – 26 mEq/L

INDICATIONS

ABG is a rapid test done to decide and direct the treatment for critically ill patients and to determine gas exchange levels in the blood as related to the respiratory system, metabolic system, and renal function.

INTERPRETATION

The ABG test gives specific information about the acid-base balance and gas exchange levels in arterial blood at specific time. It is the only way to measure the alveolar arterial gradient in the lungs. Monitoring the treatment response in mechanical ventilation.

INCREASED pH LEVELS (Alkalosis)

Metabolic alkalosis: aldosteronism, chronic vomiting, chronic gastric suction, hypochloremia, hypokalemia, mercurial diuretics.

Respiratory alkalosis: carbon monoxide poisoning, chronic heart failure, acute and severe pulmonary disease, pulmonary emboli, shock, anxiety neuroses, cystic fibrosis, pain, pregnancy.

DECREASED pH LEVELS (Acidosis)

Metabolic acidosis: ketoacidosis, renal failure, lactic acidosis, diarrhea.

Respiratory Acidosis: respiratory failure.

INCREASED Pco2 LEVELS

Chronic obstructive pulmonary disease, over oxygenation in a patient with COPD, over sedation, head trauma, Pickwickian Syndrome.

DECREASED Pco2 LEVELS

Pulmonary emboli, anxiety, hypoxemia, pain, pregnancy.

INCREASED Po2 AND INCREASED O2 CONTENT

Hyperventilation, increased inspired O2.

DECREASED Po2 AND INCREASED O2 CONTENT

Adult respiratory distress syndrome, bronchospasm, emboli, inadequate oxygen in inspired air (suffocation), pneumothorax.

Pulmonary edema, restrictive lung disease, anemias, atelectasis, atrial or ventricular cardiac septal defects, severe hypoventilation like over sedation and neurologic somnolence.

INCREASED HCO3 LEVELS

Chronic obstructive pulmonary disease, mercurial diuretics, aldosteronism, chronic and high-volume gastric suction, chronic vomiting.

DECREASED HCO3 LEVELS

Acute renal failure, chronic use of loop diuretics, diabetic ketoacidosis, starvation, chronic and severe diarrhea.

NURSING IMPLICATIONS

Monitor the respiratory rate of the patient, auscultate breath sounds, note the declining level of consciousness (GLASGOW scale), monitor heartrate and rhythm, encourage and assist with deep-breathing exercises, turning, and coughing. Administer medications as indicated. Suction should be done as necessary. Provide airway adjunct as indicated. Monitor and graph serial ABGs, pulse oximetry readings, Hb, serum electrolyte level, administer oxygen as indicated. Assist with ventilatory aids.

NOTES

_____
_____
_____
_____
_____
_____
_____
_____
_____
_____
_____

LIVER FUNCTION TESTS

L iver function blood tests are used to aid the diagnosis of liver diseases and to monitor liver damage. There are many different functions of the liver, and many different tests have been devised to measure liver function. Liver function tests are divided according to the function of the liver they measure. The major pigment in the body is the heme part of hemoglobin. When red blood cells die, the hemoglobin is liberated and the heme is separated from globin. The iron atom is removed and the porphyrin ring opened, converting the heme to biliverdin and then to bilirubin.

This bilirubin though closely bound to albumin is known as free bilirubin and is normally present in plasma or serum in very small quantities. In the liver, this free bilirubin is taken up by the hepatic cells and combined with glucuronic acid to form conjugated bilirubin. A small amount of conjugated bilirubin gets into the blood and can be detected in the serum; most of it is excreted in bile. Conjugated bilirubin is not bound to protein, and it can therefore pass through the glomerulus and appear in the urine.

Free bilirubin is poorly soluble in water whereas conjugated bilirubin is very soluble. This difference in solubility of the two forms of bilirubin allows us to distinguish between the two in the chemical procedure used to measure bilirubin in the serum. Bilirubin in the bile is reduced by bacteria in the intestine to form urobilinogen (stercobilinogen). The greater part of the urobilinogen is reabsorbed and carried back to the liver (enterohepatic circulation) and reexcreted in the bile, although a small amount escapes into the systemic circulation. The urobilinogen in the feces is oxidized to urobilin (stercobilin). These substances together make up the bile pigments.

The liver is very much a part of the metabolism of lipids. This includes synthesis, esterification (turning lipids into soluble salts), and the storage and excretion of cholesterol. The liver also plays a very important role in the metabolism of carbohydrates by the formation and storage of glycogen while it helps the breakdown of glycogen to maintain blood glucose level and the supply of glucose to cells throughout the body. The liver is also involved in protein metabolism both through the synthesis of many proteins by the hepatic cells like albumin, prothrombin, fibrinogen, and many coagulation factors and also by the synthesis of urea as the final product of protein metabolism. There are a number of enzymes present in serum found in greater levels when there is damage to hepatic cells or obstruction of bile excretion.

Certain enzymes and proteins in the blood like alanine aminotransferase, aspartate aminotransferase, bilirubin, albumin, ammonia, amylase, lipase, protein, and lipids are measured by these tests. Liver function tests are also done to monitor the normal functions of the liver like the production of protein and bilirubin clearance, a waste product of the blood. Some enzymes are released by the liver cells in response to damage or disease. Deranged levels can indicate liver diseases.

Liver function tests include:

Alanine transaminase (ALT) is an enzyme that converts proteins into energy for the liver cells. It was earlier called serum glutamic pyruvic transaminase (SGPT). A low level of ALT is normally present in the serum. Liver damage increases alanine transaminase, and ALT is also used to screen and monitor liver disease.

Aspartate transaminase (AST) is an enzyme that metabolizes amino acids. It was originally called as serum glutamic oxaloacetic transaminase (SGOT). Like ALT, AST is normally found in blood in small quantities. An elevation in AST levels may indicate liver damage, disease, or muscle damage. The enzyme is released when there is damage to these organs or hemolysis, resulting in elevated AST levels in the serum. Serum levels reflect the extent of damage.

The liver and bone contain alkaline phosphatase (ALP), an enzyme important for protein break down. In the liver, the bile ducts are lined with cells that contain ALP. Bile ducts are small tubules that drain bile from the liver to the intestine, and the ALP in these bile ductular cells helps to digest fat in the diet. Higher-than-normal levels of ALP may suggest bile duct blockage, liver damage or disease, or certain bone diseases.

Albumin is an important protein of the body and is made in the liver. These proteins fight infections, and they are needed by the body to perform other functions like modulation of plasma oncotic pressure while they help in the transport of ligands like bilirubin, ions, fatty acids and drugs. Decreased levels of albumin below the normal range may indicate liver damage or disease.

Bilirubin is a breakdown product of red blood cells. Bilirubin traverses through the liver and is excreted in the urine and stools. Jaundice is the yellowish discoloration of the skin due elevated levels of bilirubin that might indicate liver damage or disease or certain anemias. Bilirubin is a breakdown product of heme degradation. About 70%-90% of bilirubin is derived from hemoglobin degradation and from other heme proteins to a smaller extent. Both direct bilirubin (DBil) and total-value bilirubin (TBil) are measured in the serum.

Gamma-glutamyl transferase (GGT) is a liver enzyme present in the blood in small amounts. Elevated levels of GGT may suggest liver or bile duct damage.

L-lactate dehydrogenase (LD) is another one of the panel of enzymes found in the liver. Higher than normal levels may indicate liver damage but can be elevated in many other disorders.

Prothrombin time (PT) is the measure of time taken by the blood to clot. Increased PT may suggest liver damage, but it can also be elevated if patients are on anticoagulants or blood-thinning drugs, such as Coumadin.

NOTES

_____

_____

_____

_____

_____

_____

The alanine aminotransferase (ALT) test is used to detect and monitor injury to the hepatocellular component, inflammation of the liver, and to assess the improvement or worsening of the disease in response to treatment. ALT was earlier known as serum glutamic pyruvic transaminase (SGPT).

NORMAL RANGES
Adult male: 10 to 55 units/L ; Female: 7 to 30 units/L

INDICATIONS
The ALT test is done when liver disease is suspected and also to monitor the liver function.

INTERPRETATION
Alanine aminotransferase (ALT) is usually measured concurrently with AST as part of a liver function panel to determine the cause of organ damage. ALT is a primary enzyme in the liver that has a longer half-life and is more specific for liver damage, whereas AST is systemic and found in many other organs.

INCREASED LEVELS
Hepatitis, hepatic necrosis, hepatic ischemia, hepatotoxic drugs, hepatic tumor, cirrhosis, cholestasis, obstructive jaundice, pancreatitis, infectious mononucleosis, myocardial infarction, myositis, severe burns, trauma to striated muscle.

DECREASED LEVELS
is expected and normal.

INTERFERING FACTORS
Vitamin B6 depletion can show falsely low AST and ALT levels. Hemolyzed specimens should not be used for this test.

NURSING IMPLICATIONS
Patients should be informed that fasting is not required and intramuscular injections taken previously may cause elevated levels.

The aspartate aminotransferase (AST) test is used to assess and aid in diagnosis of a patient with a supposed hepatocellular disease, injury, or inflammation. Along with cardiac markers, it could also be used to evaluate coronary artery occlusive disease. AST was previously known as serum glutamic-oxaloacetic transaminase (SGOT).

NORMAL RANGES

Adult male: 10 – 40 units/L, Female: 9 – 25 units/L

INDICATIONS

The AST test is done simultaneously with ALT when liver disease or damage is suspected and also to monitor the liver function and response to treatment.

INTERPRETATION

Conditions associated with very high aspartate aminotransferase levels are liver damage in conditions like acute viral hepatitis, acute fulminant hepatitis, tumor necrosis, toxins/drugs including acetaminophen overdose.

INCREASED LEVELS

Liver diseases: drug-induced liver injury, hepatic necrosis, hepatitis, hepatic cirrhosis, hepatic metastasis, hepatic surgery, heart diseases, cardiac operations, myocardial infarctions, cardiac catheterization and angioplasty,

skeletal muscle diseases: heat stroke, progressive muscular dystrophy, multiple traumas, primary muscle diseases, recent noncardiac surgery, severe burns, acute hemolytic anemia, acute pancreatitis.

DECREASED LEVELS

Chronic renal dialysis, diabetic ketoacidosis, pregnancy, acute renal disease, beriberi.

INTERFERING FACTORS

An elevated AST and normal ALT can indicate a normal liver, but damage to other organs and/or hemolysis because ALT is found in various other organs, Vitamin B6 depletion can result in falsely low AST and ALT levels. Hemolyzed specimens should not be used.

NURSING IMPLICATIONS

Instruct the patient that fasting is not required. Elevated levels can be seen due to previous intramuscular injections.

Bilirubin is formed by the liver, spleen, and bone marrow and is a breakdown product of hemoglobin. Total bilirubin levels are further broken into direct bilirubin and indirect bilirubin. Any type of jaundice can increase the total bilirubin level. The values of direct and indirect bilirubin levels help differentiate the various causes of jaundice.

NORMAL RANGES

Bilirubin Total: 0.3 – 1.0 mg/dL, Direct bilirubin: 0.0 to 0.2 mg/dL, Indirect bilirubin: 0.1 to 1 mg/dL, critical level: > 12 mg/dL

INDICATIONS

The bilirubin test is done in suspected liver disease and also to monitor the liver function.

INTERPRETATION

Higher than normal levels of bilirubin indicate liver damage. Elevated direct bilirubin indicates that the liver is not clearing the bilirubin properly.

INCREASED LEVELS

Extrahepatic duct obstruction (inflammation, scarring, surgical trauma, or tumor), cholestasis from drugs, Dubin-Johnson syndrome, extensive liver metastasis, gallstones, Rotor's Syndrome.

DECREASED LEVELS

Erythroblastosis fetalis, Gilbert's Syndrome, cirrhosis, Crigler-Najjar Syndrome, hemolytic jaundice, hepatitis, neonatal hyperbilirubinemia, hematoma, pernicious anemia, sepsis, transfusion reaction.

INTERFERING FACTORS

The results will be elevated with the ingestion of alcohol or the administration of theophylline, ascorbic acid (vitamin C), morphine sulfate, or acetylsalicylic acid (aspirin).

NURSING IMPLICATIONS

The patient should be told to eat a diet low in yellow foods, avoiding foods such as carrots, yellow beans, and pumpkin for 3 to 4 days before the blood is drawn. The test requires fasting for 4 hours before the blood sample is drawn. If the patient has received a radioactive scan within 24 hours prior to the test, the results are invalid.

Albumin is the most important protein of the blood that regulates plasma oncotic pressure and transports ligands endogenous ligands like bilirubin, fatty acids, hormones and exogenous ligands like drugs and other substances that are insoluble in water.

NORMAL RANGE
3.4 to 5 g/dL

INDICATIONS
Albumin is decreased in conditions such as acute infection, ascites, and alcoholism and increased in conditions such as dehydration, diarrhea, and metastatic carcinoma. If albumin, or protein, is detected in the urine it is indicative of abnormal renal function.

INTERPRETATION
Albumin testing is done to identify if the body is not absorbing enough protein or if the patient has liver or kidney disease.

INCREASED LEVELS
Dehydration, severe diarrhea, severe vomiting.

DECREASED LEVELS
Acute liver failure, increased capillary permeability, malnutrition, pregnancy, cirrhosis, familial idiopathic dysproteinemia protein-losing enteropathies, protein-losing nephropathies, inflammatory disease, severe burns, severe malnutrition, ulcerative colitis.

INTERFERING FACTORS
Anabolic steroids, androgens, growth hormones and insulin interfere with the measurement of albumin. Marked lipemia can interfere with albumin measurement. Albumin is decreased in the third trimester of pregnancy; Large amounts of intravenous fluids may give inaccurate results.

NURSING IMPLICATIONS
No fasting is indicated

Ammonia is formed as a by-product of protein catabolism. It is generated in the gut by the action of proteins on the bacteria normally present. Metabolism of ammonia takes place in the liver and is excreted by the kidneys as urea. When there is hepatic dysfunction, elevated levels of ammonia may lead to encephalopathy.

NORMAL RANGE

Adults: 35 – 65 mcg/dL

INDICATIONS

This test, is used to assure the diagnosis of Reye Syndrome or hepatic encephalopathy caused by liver disease which results in changes in behavior and consciousness, to investigate the cause of coma of unexplainable origin, and to evaluate a urea cycle defect.

INTERPRETATION

Increased ammonia in circulation causes hyperbilirubinemia by inhibiting cell growth, causing apoptosis and damages the mitochondria of the hepatocytes. Therefore, energy synthesis is reduced, which in turn reduces the expression of enzymes associated with bilirubin metabolism.

INCREASED LEVELS

Reye Syndrome, Liver disease, cirrhosis, hepatic coma, Inherited urea cycle defect, hemolytic disease in infants (erythroblastosis fetalis), renal disease, certain inborn errors of metabolism of urea Gastrointestinal (GI) hemorrhage.

DECREASED LEVELS

Hyperornithinemia, hypothyroidism, essential or malignant hypertension, Use of certain antibiotics (e.g. neomycin).

INTERFERING FACTORS

High glucose levels, hemolysis. Smoking is toxic and increases ammonia levels.

NURSING IMPLICATIONS

The patient should fast except for water. The patient should avoid smoking for 8 to 10 hours before the test. The sample should not be hemolyzed. The specimen should be sent promptly to the laboratory for analysis. High glucose levels over 500 mg/dL may interfere with the test.

Amylase is one of the enzymes produced by the pancreas and salivary glands. These enzymes help in the breakdown and digestion of complex carbohydrates and are excreted by the kidneys. They convert starch into maltose, and further enzymes in the small intestine convert them into monosaccharides.

NORMAL RANGES

25 to 151 units/L

INDICATIONS

Amylase is measured in conjunction with a lipase test to diagnose acute pancreatitis and to monitor other pancreatic disorders.

INTERPRETATION

Acute pancreatitis is an emergency and comes with intense pain where the amylase level may exceed five times the normal value. It starts increasing in 6 hours after the onset of pain, peaks at about 24 hours, and takes 2 to 3 days to return to normal after the onset of pain. In chronic pancreatitis, the serum amylase level increases but not more than three times the normal value.

INCREASED LEVELS

Acute pancreatitis, acute cholecystitis, parotitis, peptic ulcer, duodenal obstruction, diabetic ketoacidosis, ectopic pregnancy, necrotic bowel, perforated bowel, pulmonary infarction.

DECREASED LEVELS

Chronic pancreatitis, liver disease, cystic fibrosis, preeclampsia

INTERFERING FACTORS

Drugs containing asparaginase, birth control pills, aspirin.

NURSING IMPLICATIONS

On the laboratory form, make a list of the medications that the patient has taken during the previous 24 hours before the test. If the specimen was obtained after cholecystography within 72 hours of the procedure where radiopaque dyes are used, the results are invalidated.

Lipase is a pancreatic enzyme that converts fats and triglycerides into fatty acids and glycerol. Pancreatic disorders show elevated lipase levels. Elevations take 24 to 36 hours to occur after the onset of illness and may remain elevated for up to 14 days.

NORMAL RANGES
10 to 140 units/L

INDICATIONS
The lipase test is done along with amylase in acute pancreatitis. It is also used in the diagnosis of peritonitis, strangulated or infarcted bowel, and pancreatic cyst.

INTERPRETATION
In acute alcoholic pancreatitis, lipase levels remain elevated longer than amylase and, therefore, its sensitivity is increased. Hence, serum lipase may be a more reliable indicator than serum amylase for the initial diagnosis of acute pancreatitis.

INCREASED LEVELS
Acute pancreatitis, chronic relapsing pancreatitis, extrahepatic duct obstruction, pancreatic cancer, pancreatic pseudocyst, acute cholecystitis, bowel obstruction or infarction, cholangitis, peptic ulcer disease, renal failure.

DECREASED LEVELS
Chronic conditions such as cystic fibrosis.

INTERFERING FACTORS
The presence of hemoglobin, quinine, heavy metals, calcium ions decrease the lipase levels.

NURSING IMPLICATIONS
Endoscopic retrograde cholangiopancreatography (ERCP) increases lipase activity.

Serum protein gives a measure of the total amount of albumin and globulins in the plasma. Proteins form a major component of blood, skin, hair, nails, and internal organs.

NORMAL RANGE

6 to 8 g/dL

INDICATIONS

The patient's overall nutritional status is obtained by the assessment of serum protein levels, especially if the patient comes with a history of unknown cause of significant weight loss. This test is also indicated to assess liver disorders, renal disorders, and bone marrow disorders as part of liver function tests, and to investigate the cause of edema.

INTERPRETATION

Protein is responsible for regulating plasma oncotic pressure and is necessary for the formation of many hormones, enzymes, and antibodies.

INCREASED LEVELS

chronic infection, Crohn's disease, hepatitis B, hepatitis C, Addison's disease, autoimmune collagen disorders, amyloidosis, dehydration, human immunodeficiency virus, multiple myeloma.

DECREASED LEVELS

Kidney disorder, liver disease, severe malnutrition, agammaglobulinemia, bleeding, celiac disease, extensive burns, inflammatory bowel disease.

INTERFERING FACTORS

Drugs like allopurinol, asparaginase, azathioprine, chlorpropamide, cisplatin, dapsone, dextran, estrogens, ibuprofen, progesterone, acute and chronic inflammations and decreased liver synthesis, albumin values normally decrease in third trimester of pregnancy.

NURSING IMPLICATIONS

Make a list of medications the patient is taking, Inform the patient about the test procedure. No fluid or food restrictions are required before the procedure.

LIPID PROFILE

E nergy is stored in the body in the form of triglycerides, the most abundant dietary lipid compound found throughout the diet. The liver is a part of lipid metabolism which includes formation, esterification to convert lipid into a soluble salt, storage and the excretion of cholesterol. Cholesterol is a vital component of a cell membrane and a precursor of the synthesis of bile salts and steroid hormones. Since the liver is so involved in the metabolism of cholesterol, it is easy to understand how levels in the serum will vary in liver disease. Where there is injury or destruction of hepatic cells, as in viral hepatitis, the level of cholesterol is often decreased. In severe hepatitis and cirrhosis, the level is also often decreased. But when there is obstruction to the bile flow from the liver, serum cholesterol may be elevated.

Inherited abnormalities of cholesterol metabolism are rare. Measurement of cholesterol levels as one gets older is important because high serum cholesterol levels are indicative of a high risk for cardiovascular disease. Serum cholesterol levels can usually be lowered by less fat and dairy product consumption in the diet. Serum cholesterol levels are also found to be elevated in hypothyroidism and nephrotic syndrome.

Pancreatic lipase digests dietary triglycerides initially. Once the cholecystokinin is released, bile salts are released in the duodenum in response. Lipid micelles are formed by bile salts, which form a hydrophobic core of lipid molecules and a hydrophilic surface, including FFA.

Lipid compounds get absorbed into cells through diffusion into the enterocyte for biochemical use and also get transported through lipid transporters located on the luminal side of the enterocyte. After they enter the enterocyte, they form into triglycerides and are packaged by the Golgi apparatus into chylomicrons to receive chylomicron specific apolipoproteins, called apo B48, which is a marker for TG chylomicron. The enterocyte then releases the chylomicrons and enters circulation by the lymphatic system.

The triglyceride-rich chylomicrons, once in circulation, pass through the vasculature and undergo protein exchange, a complex process mediated by HDL.

Based on this exchange, they either undergo dilapidation on the vascular endothelial surface by lipoprotein lipase (LPL) or are received in the liver for further metabolism and packaging. Triglycerides are packaged into very-low dense lipoprotein (VLDL) for transport to peripheral tissues. In short, they are formed from triglycerides that undergo hepatic uptake.

Thus, the major carrier of triglycerides and FFA in the serum is VLDL synthesized within the hepatocyte. A smaller percentage of FFA is complexed to albumin for transport and travels in an unesterified form. After the VLDL is released into serum, it traverses to the peripheral tissues where it undergoes a dilapidation cascade, and the triglyceride is removed by LPL at LPL receptor sites along the endothelium. After the process of dilapidation, a VLDL remnant (IDL) is formed by shedding the bulk of the triglyceride and is cleared by the liver or transformed to LDL by a serum protein exchange process.

The major high-energy compound is the triglyceride, which stores energy and supplies 9 Kcal/g of free fatty acid. Triglycerides and FFA have a major role in the etiopathogenesis of atherosclerotic disease formation. Elevated levels of atherogenic lipoproteins use high triglycerides that contain triglyceride and FFA as a marker. Elevated triglycerides also indicate insulin resistance in the presence of low levels of HDL and elevated LDL. Patients with this lipid profile are at a high risk for coronary heart disease. A major clinical risk factor for coronary artery disease (CAD) is hypercholesterolemia, especially hypertriglyceridemia, especially when the HDL levels are low.

NOTES

_____
_____
_____
_____
_____
_____
_____
_____

A lipoprotein assessment or lipid profile includes total cholesterol, high-density lipoprotein (HDL), low-density lipoprotein (LDL), and triglycerides. Cholesterol is a major component of LDL that is present in all body tissues, cell membranes, brain, nerve cells, and some gallstones.

Triglycerides constitute a small part of LDLs and a major part of very-low-density lipoproteins (VLDL). Increased triglyceride levels, cholesterol levels and LDL levels put the patient at a high risk for coronary artery disease. High LDL increases the risk and high HDL protects against the risk of coronary artery disease.

NORMAL RANGES

Cholesterol < 200 mg/dL, Triglycerides < 150 mg/dL, HDLs: 30 to 70 mg/dL, LDLs < 130 mg/dL

INDICATIONS

Both men and women are at an equally increased risk for coronary artery disease. Males aged 35 years and older and females aged 45 years and older should undergo lipid profile screening. Screening of blood cholesterol levels in children and adolescents is recommended for children in families where familial dyslipidemias and premature heart ailments has been established.

INTERPRETATION

Normal values of triglycerides (TG) should be less than 150mg/dL. Elevated triglycerides are serum blood values being greater than 149mg/dL. Very high serum levels of triglycerides of more than 500mg/dL can cause development of acute pancreatitis.

INCREASED HDL LEVELS

Familial HDL lipoproteinemia, extensive exercise.

DECREASED HDL LEVELS

Familial low HDL, hypoproteinemia in malnutrition or nephrotic syndrome, hepatocellular disease like cirrhosis or hepatitis, metabolic syndrome.

INCREASED LDL AND VLDL LEVELS

Familial LDL lipoproteinemia, familial hypercholesterolemia type IIa gammopathies like multiple myeloma, alcohol consumption, apoprotein CII deficiency, chronic liver disease, Cushing's Syndrome, glycogen storage diseases like von Gierke's disease, hepatoma, hypothyroidism, nephrotic syndrome.

DECREASED LDL AND VLDL LEVELS

Hypoproteinemia in severe burns, malnutrition or malabsorption, familial hypolipoproteinemia, hyperthyroidism.

INTERFERING FACTORS

Patients who have consumed a meal rich in lipid compounds and have not fasted for 8 hours prior to venipuncture can show false positive high-triglyceride levels in the screening lipid panels. Alcoholics can show elevated triglycerides in the serum.

NURSING IMPLICATIONS

Oral contraceptives may increase the lipid level, patients should fast and avoid foods and fluids, except water, for 12 to 14 hours. Patients should not consume alcohol for 24 hours before the test. Patients should not eat high-cholesterol foods with dinner before the morning sample is drawn for the test.

NOTES

_____

_____

_____

_____

_____

_____

_____

_____

_____

_____

CARDIAC MARKERS AND SERUM ENZYMES

C ardiac markers and enzymes are intracellular components that can be measured in the serum under certain circumstances like trauma, myocardial ischemia, and myocarditis. Myocardial injury causes a release of serum enzymes and cardiac markers into circulation as seen in myocardial infarction (MI) or other diseases of the heart, such as heart failure.

In suspected acute coronary syndrome (ACS), cardiac markers and enzymes are used in the diagnosis and stratification of risk in patients with chest pain. Cardiac troponins are the first choice of cardiac markers in patients with ACS.

The guidelines from the European Society of Cardiology (ESC) and the American College of Cardiology (ACC) have made cardiac troponin central to the definition of acute myocardial infarction (MI). Cardiac troponins have superior sensitivity and accuracy; and the guidelines suggest that cardiac biomarkers should be verified at presentation in patients with suspected MI. It is the only biomarker recommended for diagnosis in myocardial infarction. Acute MI shows an early elevated troponin level within 2-3 hours of hospital arrival in 80% of cases, whereas CK-MB and other cardiac markers are elevated at 6-9 hours or more. Moreover, with atypical presentations, serum cardiac enzymes can become the only correct method of identifying problems.

For diagnosis of patients who present with ischemic chest pain and diagnostic ST-segment elevation in the electrocardiogram, evaluation of cardiac markers is not required. These patients may need to undergo thrombolytic therapy or primary angioplasty. Since the sensitivity of cardiac markers is low in the first 6 hours after the onset of symptoms, treatment should not be delayed by waiting for cardiac marker results. Immediate reperfusion therapy for patients with ST-segment elevation MI (STEMI), without waiting for cardiac marker results, is recommended by the American Heart Association (AHA).

Troponins are found in skeletal and cardiac muscle; they are regulatory proteins Three subunits of troponin have been identified: troponin I (TnI), troponin T (TnT), and troponin C (TnC). The skeletal and cardiac subforms for TnI and troponin TnT are very specific and distinct; and various immunoassays have been made to differentiate them.

Earlier, the biochemical marker of choice for the diagnosis of acute MI was the CK-MB isoenzyme before the recommendation for troponins came in. Two serial elevations of CK-MB above the diagnostic cutoff level or a single elevated result twice the value of the upper limit was considered the diagnostic criteria for acute MI. Although the CK-MB is concentrated in the heart muscle, CK-MB also exists in skeletal muscle, resulting in a number of false-positive elevations in many clinical settings, including myopathy, trauma and heavy exertion.

CK-MB first appears in the serum 4-6 hours after the onset of symptoms and peaks at 24 hours. It then returns to normal in 48-72 hours. One of the earliest markers of MI is myoglobin, a heme protein found in skeletal and cardiac muscle. It has attracted considerable repute as an early marker of MI. Its early release profile is attributed to its low molecular weight, and it typically elevates within 2-4 hours after onset of infarction, then peaks at 6-12 hours before returning to normal within 24-36 hours.

Rapid myoglobin assays have become available, but they lack cardio specificity. Therefore, serial sampling is recommended every 1-2 hours which increases sensitivity and specificity. An increase of 25-40% over 1-2 hours is strongly suggestive of acute MI. According to many studies, myoglobin only achieved 90% sensitivity for acute MI , so the negative predictive value of myoglobin is not high enough, and it cannot exclude the diagnosis of acute MI.

The enzyme creatine kinase (CK) is found in heart, muscle, and brain tissue that reflects tissue catabolism resulting from cell trauma. The creatinine kinase level begins to increase within 6 hours of damage to the muscle and reaches the peak at 18 hours before returning to normal in 2 to 3 days.

NORMAL LAB VALUES OF CREATININE KINASE AND ISOENZYMES
Creatinine kinase (CK):
Women: 26 – 140 U/L
Men: 38 – 174 U/L, isoenzymes of creatinine kinase: CK-MM: 95% – 100% of total, CK-MB: 0% – 5% of total, CK-BB: 0%

INDICATIONS
The test for CK is done to assess myocardial damage and central nervous system damage or skeletal muscle damage. Isoenzymes of creatinine kinase include CK-MB (cardiac muscle), CK-BB (brain), and CK-MM (muscles):

- CK-MM is found in skeletal muscle mainly.
- CK-MB is found mainly in cardiac muscle.
- CK-BB is found in brain tissue.

INTERPRETATION
Increased creatinine kinase is commonly used to aid the diagnosis of acute myocardial infarction and neuromuscular diseases. Neuromuscular disorders which show elevated CK enzymes are myopathies, rhabdomyolysis, malignant hyperthermia, muscular dystrophy, drug-induced myopathies, neuroleptic malignant syndrome, and periodic paralyses.

INCREASED LEVELS OF CPK-BB ISOENZYME
Adenocarcinoma of breast and lungs, central nervous system diseases, pulmonary infarction.

INCREASED LEVELS OF CPK -MB ISOENZYME
Acute myocardial infarction, myocarditis, cardiac aneurysm surgery, cardiac defibrillation, cardiac ischemia, ventricular arrhythmias.

INCREASED LEVELS OF CPK -MM ISOENZYME
Muscular dystrophy, myositis, crush injuries, malignant hyperthermia, recent convulsions, recent surgery, delirium tremens, electroconvulsive therapy, electromyography, hypokalemia, hypothyroidism, IM injections, rhabdomyolysis, shock, trauma.

INTERFERING FACTORS

Intramuscular injections and invasive procedures may falsely elevate CK levels.

NURSING IMPLICATIONS

Strenuous physical activity should be avoided by the patient for 24 hours prior to the test if it is for skeletal muscle. The patient should also avoid ingestion of alcohol for 24 hours prior to the test.

NOTES

_____
_____
_____
_____
_____
_____
_____
_____
_____
_____
_____
_____
_____
_____
_____
_____
_____
_____
_____
_____
_____
_____
_____

A protein called myoglobin is found in the striated (cardiac and skeletal) muscle. It binds to oxygen and releases oxygen at very low tensions. Myoglobin is released into the blood whenever there is injury to the skeletal muscle. Myoglobin rises 2-4 hours after an MI; hence it is used as an early marker for determining cardiac damage.

NORMAL RANGES
5–70 ng/mL

INDICATIONS
Early myocardial infarction shows a rise in the myoglobin as early as 2-4 hours. it is also elevated following muscle injury and in inflammatory and degenerative muscle diseases.

INTERPRETATION
Serum myoglobin levels show a rise within two to three hours following a myocardial infarction. These levels reach their highest values within 8 to 12 hours. Myoglobin levels return to normal levels within 24 hours.

INCREASED LEVELS
Myocardial infarction, rhabdomyolysis, skeletal muscle ischemia, skeletal muscle trauma, myositis, malignant hyperthermia, muscular dystrophy.

INTERFERING FACTORS
A recent angina attack may show increased myoglobin levels. Increased myoglobin levels are also seen in cardioversion, kidney disease, heavy alcohol consumption and the use of certain drugs.

NURSING IMPLICATIONS
The myoglobin level can increase within 2 hours after a myocardial infarction, and shows a rapid fall in the level after 7 hours. As the myoglobin level gets elevated in skeletal muscle conditions, it is not cardiac specific. It also rises and falls rapidly, making its use limited in diagnosing myocardial infarction.

Troponin is a regulatory protein found in myocardial and skeletal striated muscle. When an infarction results in damage to the myocardium, increased amounts of troponin are released into the bloodstream.

NORMAL RANGES

Troponin: Lesser than 0.04 ng/mL; value above 0.40 ng/mL indicates myocardial infarction

Troponin I: Lesser than 0.6 ng/mL; value above1.5 ng/mL is indicative of myocardial infarction

Troponin T: More than 0.1 to 0.2 ng/mL is indicative of myocardial infarction

INDICATIONS

Troponins are the most important enzymes released in response to myocardial injury, regardless of the cause. Myocardial ischemia leading to infarction is the most common cause of cardiac muscle damage. Serial measurements of troponin are recommended to compare with baseline test results. Troponin enzyme elevations are specific and clinically significant in the diagnosis of heart pathology.

INTERPRETATION

Troponin levels begin to increase as early as 3 hours after Myocardial infarction. Troponin I levels may remain elevated for 7 to 10 days and troponin T levels may remain elevated for about 10 to 14 days.

INCREASED LEVELS

Myocardial infarction, myocarditis, pericarditis, cardiac contusion/trauma, myocardial injury, endocarditis, cardiac surgery, pulmonary embolism, aortic dissection.

INTERFERING FACTORS

Drugs with cardiotoxic properties may also elevate troponins. Most commonly, they are chemicals such as carbon monoxide and chemotherapeutic drugs such as cyclophosphamide, anthracyclines, and bevacizumab.

NURSING IMPLICATIONS

Change venipuncture sites. Serial testing is advised and repeated in 12 hours or as prescribed. It is then followed by daily testing for 3 to 5 days.

Natriuretic peptides are neuroendocrine peptides used as markers for patients in heart failure. There are three major peptides:

- Atrial natriuretic peptides (ANP) secreted in cardiac atrial muscle
- Brain natriuretic peptides (BNP) secreted in the cardiac ventricular muscle
- C-type natriuretic peptides (CNP) secreted by endothelial cells

NORMAL RANGES

Atrial natriuretic peptide (ANP): From 22 to 27 pg/mL;
Brain natriuretic peptide (BNP) less than 100 pg/mL; C-type natriuretic peptide (CNP).Results should be reviewed with the reference range provided.

INDICATIONS

To identify heart failure as the cause of dyspnea, the BNP is used as the primary marker. The higher the Brain natriuretic peptides level, the more severe the heart failure. If the BNP is normal, the dyspnea is due to a pulmonary problem; and if the Brain natriuretic peptides level is elevated, dyspnea is due to heart failure.

INTERPRETATION

In an acutely dyspneic patient, a BNP value of < 100 pg/mL makes the diagnosis of congestive heart failure less likely. Elevated levels of natriuretic peptides are indicative of poor long term prognosis in coronary artery disease, congestive heart failure, and atrial fibrillation.

INCREASED LEVELS

Systemic hypertension Congestive heart failure, cor pulmonale, heart transplant rejection, myocardial infarction.

INTERFERING FACTORS

False low levels: obesity, pulmonary edema. False high levels: females, advancing age, renal failure.

NURSING IMPLICATIONS

There is no necessity of fasting for this test.

HIV AND AIDS TESTING

Human immunodeficiency virus is blood borne and sexually transmissible. This virus weakens immunity by attacking the most important cells that defend against viruses. The route of transmission is by sexual intercourse, shared intravenous drug syringes and other material, and vertical transmission from a mother-to-child (MTCT), which can occur during delivery or during breastfeeding. The body fluids that transmit this disease are semen, saliva, blood, vaginal fluids, rectal fluids, and breastmilk.

The transmission route is different in various populations and depends on the introduction of the virus initially and also local practices. Other viruses transmitted by similar routes are hepatitis B, hepatitis C, and human herpesvirus 8, also known as Kaposi sarcoma herpes virus [KSHV]). These viruses can cause a coinfection in HIV infected patients.

HIV-1 and HIV-2 are the two distinct types HIV; each is composed of several subtypes. HIV-1 and HIV-2 appear similar, but they are made of unique genes and have their own process of replication.

The CDC guidelines recommend that everyone between the age of 13 and 64 get tested as a part of routine health care. Getting tested early in the disease and taking medications reduces the viral load of HIV effectively and increases expected survival.

The HIV-2 virus carries a lesser risk of transmission and progresses more slowly to acquired immune deficiency syndrome (AIDS). The viral load in HIV-2 is less than people with HIV-1, where the viral load is higher, and there is rapid progression to AIDS in HIV-1 infections.

A lot of negative attitudes or stigmas have been attached to HIV infection, mostly because of the sexually transmitted route of the virus and the inference of sexual promiscuity. There is also prejudice that an infected individual or group is socially unacceptable. This stigma has led to reluctance to be tested for HIV infection and also disrupts the emotional well-being and mental health of the individual. It has resulted in the refusal to have casual contact with HIV infected individuals. The HIV virus isn't transmitted by casual contact and is inactivated by use of simple detergents. The concern with HIV is the continuous decline in the immune system and the incurability of the infection, leading to premature death in the majority of infected people.

Common tests used to look for the presence of antibodies to HIV include ELISA, immunofluorescence assay (IFA) and Western blot, which assess the nucleic acids, antigen/antibody or antibody tests. A single reactive ELISA test is not enough to diagnose HIV and should be repeated with the same blood sample. If the test is reactive again, follow-up tests should be done with Western blot or IFA. HIV is confirmed by a positive Western blot or IFA result. If the treatment is started immediately after the patient is diagnosed with HIV, it reduces the viral load and helps reduce the progression of the disease and protects the immune system.

If the viral load is not detectable in the blood due to antiretroviral therapy in HIV, the risk of transmission is reduced drastically. Being HIV positive doesn't mean that the patient has AIDS. If a person diagnosed with HIV takes treatment as prescribed, the patient may stay healthy for many years and may not be diagnosed with AIDS at all.

NOTES

_____
_____
_____
_____
_____
_____
_____
_____
_____
_____
_____
_____

The pathogenesis of HIV is largely because of the decline in CD4+ T-cell counts, and it helps to monitor the progression of HIV. The decrease in immunity is also attributed to the reduction in CD4+ count. CD4+ T-cell counts higher than 500 cells/L are required to maintain a healthy immune system. When the CD4+ T-cell count is among 200 and 499 cells/L, it causes immune related problems while severe immune system problems occur when the CD4+ T-cell count is lesser than 200 cells/L.

NORMAL RANGES

Normal: 500 to 1600 cells/L

Severe: Less than 200 cells/L

CD4-to-CD8 ratio: 2:1

INDICATIONS

HIV attacks the CD4 cells responsible for immunity. If the CD4 cell count is low, the immune system of the body cannot fight and defend against infections. The range of CD4+ T cell count helps to identify the risk of complications in patients with HIV.

INTERPRETATION

CD4+ cell baseline counts have to be measured in patients with HIV every 3 to 6 months during the first 2 years. The CD4 count should be measured till it increases above 300 cells/mm3.

INCREASED LEVELS

T-cell lymphoma, B-cell lymphoma, chronic lymphocytic leukemia.

DECREASED LEVELS

HIV-positive patients, organ transplants, congenital immunodeficiency.

NURSING IMPLICATIONS

Fasting is not required before the test.

THYROID STUDIES

L aboratory tests such as thyroxine, T3, T4, and TSH assess thyroid function. Thyroid studies are evaluated if a disorder is suspected. The function of thyroid is crucial for the normal development of the fetus and to maintain a normal metabolic function. Serum levels of thyroid hormones are used
to assess the function.

Thyroid abnormalities are commonly due to an abnormal function or growth
of the gland. Hyperthyroidism or hypothyroidism present with signs and
symptoms when the levels of thyroid hormones are deranged and reflected
in the blood level of these hormones, most specifically TSH. TSH is produced
and secreted by the pituitary gland. TSH levels are the first line of testing in
assessing thyroid status, whether normal (euthyroid), hyperfunctioning (hy-
perthyroid), or hypofunctioning (hypothyroid). The pituitary-hypothalamus
axis functions on the principle of negative feedback and controls and regulates the release and production of thyroid hormones through the thyroid
gland.

The release of TSH is further controlled by the negative feedback mechanism
of thyrotropin-releasing hormone (TRH), which is secreted by the hypothalamus. TSH release is elevated when hormone levels are low and decreased
when thyroid hormone levels are high.

Primary thyroid disorders, hyperthyroidism or hypothyroidism, result from
disease in the gland itself. They are caused by the absence or deficiency of
processing enzymes or an autoimmune process attacking the cellular archi-
tecture of the gland or processing enzymes. Hyperthyroidism occurs with excess production of thyroid hormones which results in a hypermetabolic clinical and biochemical state. It is due to impaired uptake and processing of iodine due to drugs or a deficiency in the intake of thyroid hormones as in en-
demic goiter.

The disease and/or dysfunction of the pituitary or hypothalamus, leading to abnormal stimulation of the thyroid gland, results in secondary hyperthyroidism or hypothyroidism results. Goiter is an enlargement of the thyroid gland, which may or may not occur with hyperthyroidism or hypothyroidism.

In Hashimoto thyroiditis, thyroid gland enlargement is seen due to TSH stimulation caused by hypothyroidism. Hyperthyroidism is more frequent in females, showing increased levels of both T3 and T4. A toxic nodule may cause sole elevation of T3 called T3 toxicosis and is generally seen in elderly individuals.

The symptoms and signs of hyperthyroidism include weight loss, increased sweating, fatigue, insomnia, tremors, palpitations, eye changes, intolerance to heat and/or light, anxiety, tachycardia, loose motions, oligomenorrhea, infertility, and osteoporosis. The symptoms of hypothyroidism are dry hair, hair loss, myxedema, mucosal thickening causing hoarse voice, psychomotor retardation and the opposite of signs and the symptoms of hyperthyroidism mentioned above.

The enzyme-linked immunosorbent assay (ELISA) is the most common method for the estimation of T3 .

NOTES

_____

_____

_____

_____

_____

_____

_____

_____

_____

Thyroid studies are done to identify primary thyroid disease and differentiate them from secondary causes. Thyroid peroxidase antibodies detect autoimmune conditions of the thyroid gland.

NORMAL RANGES

Triiodothyronine (T_3): 80 to 230 ng/dL

Thyroxine (T_4): 5 to 12 mcg/dL

Free thyroxine (FT_4): 0.8 to 2.4 ng/dL

Thyroid-stimulating hormone or thyrotropin: 0.2 to 5.4 microunits/mL

INDICATIONS

Thyroid studies are performed if a primary thyroid disorder is suspected and also to identify secondary causes of derangement of thyroid hormone levels.

INCREASED T3 (TRIIODOTHYRONINE) LEVELS

Grave's disease, acute thyroiditis, factitious hyperthyroidism, congenital hyperproteinemia, toxic thyroid adenoma, hepatitis, pregnancy, Plummer's disease, struma ovarii.

DECREASED T3 TRIIODOTHYRONINE) LEVELS

Hypothyroidism, iodine insufficiency, hypothalamic failure, pituitary insufficiency, thyroid surgical ablation, cirrhosis, cretinism, Cushing's Syndrome, liver disease, myxedema, protein malnutrition and other protein-depleted states, renal failure.

INCREASED T4 (THYROXINE) LEVELS

Grave's disease, acute thyroiditis, familial dysalbuminemic hyperthyroxinemia, factitious hyperthyroidism, toxic thyroid adenoma, congenital hyperproteinemia, hepatitis, Pregnancy, Plummer's disease, struma ovarii.

DECREASED T4 (THYROXINE) LEVELS

Iodine insufficiency, myxedema, surgical ablation, pituitary insufficiency, cirrhosis, cretinism, Cushing's Syndrome, hypothalamic failure, protein depleted states, renal failure.

INCREASED FREE T4 (FREE THYROXINE) LEVELS

Grave's disease, toxic thyroid adenoma, acute thyroiditis, familial dysalbu-minemic, hyperthyroxinemia, congenital hyperproteinemia, factitious hy-perthyroidism, hepatitis, pregnancy, Plummer's disease, struma ovarii.

DECREASED FREE T4 (FREE THYROXINE) LEVELS

Iodine insufficiency, surgical ablation cirrhosis, hypothalamic failure, myxe-dema, cretinism, Cushing's Syndrome, pituitary insufficiency, protein-de-pleted states, renal failure.

ABNORMAL THYROID STIMULATING HORMONE (TSH) LEVELS

Hyperthyroidism, hypothyroidism, acute starvation, old age, psychiatric pri-mary depression, pregnancy.

INTERFERING FACTORS

Drugs like estrogen and biotin interfere with the thyroid function tests

NURSING IMPLICATIONS

If the patient has undergone a radionuclide scan within 7 days before the test, the results may be invalid.

NOTES

_____

_____

_____

_____

_____

_____

_____

_____

_____

_____

URINE ANALYSIS

A urine analysis is conducted for numerous reasons. Urine is one of the most simple obtainable specimens that is analyzed in the lab. The examination of urine provides information about the functioning of the kidneys and abnormalities of the urinary tract. It may also conduct to a diagnosis of many systemic illnesses of the body reflected by the existance of various substances in the urine. It is most commonly done when clinicians suspect an infection in the urinary tract and to evaluate for kidney and metabolic disorders. The test is done for both screening and diagnosis.

Urine is formed in the kidneys, the product of the ultrafiltration of plasma by the renal glomeruli, followed by reabsorption of most of the water and some of the solutes in the tubules, as well as by active secretion of some substances by the tubular epithelium. Urine is collected and passed on from the kidneys through the ureters for temporary storage in the bladder, pending final passage to the outside of the body through the urethra. The kidneys, through the functioning of the many nephron units, have the ability to selectively rid the body of many of the waste products of metabolism, while retaining essential substances, and in the process, they also regulate both water and electrolyte balance as well as the acid-base balance of the body.

COLLECTION OF URINE:

For routine examination, any fresh sample of urine is sufficient. An early morning sample is best voided when the patient arises from a night's sleep because it is the most concentrated specimen and has the lowest pH. This tends to preserve the formed elements well. For quantitative tests, a 24 hour specimen is required.

Specimens for bacteriological examination should be collected with utmost care to prevent contamination. Collection by catheterization (insertion of a sterile tube or catheter through the urethra into the bladder) into sterile containers is best when urine is needed for a culture. However, catheterization carries the risk of introducing bacteria or other infectious organisms into the urinary tract when they may not have been there in the first place. Therefore, most often urine for bacteriological examination is collected in "mid-stream" after the glans penis in the male or the anterior vulva in the female have been carefully cleaned and without touching the lip of the container to the skin surface. This is a so-called a "clean catch specimen".

It is important to instruct the patient clearly regarding the type of specimen required, especially if it is a 24 hour specimen. The early morning urine is discarded and then all urine is voided in the next 24 hours, including the early morning specimen which the next day is collected.

The containers for urine for a culture should, of course, be sterilized, and the container for the 24 urine has to be quite large, sufficient to hold at least 2 liters.

PRESERVATION OF URINE:

The urine specimen must be examined within 30-60 minutes after the patient voids to get accurate results. If there is a tentative delay in examination, the specimen should be refrigerated, though this may lead to the formation and precipitation of crystals which were in the solution at body or room temperature. A variety of preservatives are available, namely, toluene, boric acid, concentrated hydrochloric acid, formalin or chloroform, and thymol preservatives.

The urine specimen is analyzed in three phases; hence the specimen is divided into 3 parts. First, a gross visual inspection or macroscopic examination of the urine is done to determine color and clarity/turbidity of the specimen. Second, a chemical analysis is done on the specimen using a urine dipstick. The dipstick test is performed on the uncentrifuged specimen of urine, but it can also be performed after centrifugation on the supernatant.

The urine should be subjected to centrifugation at 3000 rpm for 3-5 minutes, and the supernatant is transferred in a separate tube. Strips of the reagent are dipped into the urine and compared with controls to determine urine pH, specific gravity, blood, protein, glucose, ketones, nitrites, leukocyte esterase, bilirubin, and urobilirubin.

Third, the urine is analyzed under a microscope. If centrifugation is done for microscopy, the supernatant is poured off. The sediment is resuspended and a tiny amount of the sediment is poured onto a microscopy slide. The urine sediment is then examined for elements such as cells, casts, crystals, bacteria, and yeast under the microscope. These elements in the sediment are observed as number per a high or low-power field.

URINE ANALYSIS

Color: pale yellow
Turbidity: clear
Specific gravity: 1.016 to 1.022
Odor: aromatic odor
pH: 4.5 to 7.8
Glucose: >0.5 g/day
Protein: negative
Ketones: negative
Bilirubin: negative
White blood cells: < or = 4 cells per high power field
Red blood cells: < 3 cells per high power field
Bacteria: none or >1000/ml
Crystals: none
Casts: none to few
Magnesia: 7.3 – 12.2 mg/dL
Sodium: 40 to 220 mEq/24 hours
Potassium: 25 to 125 mEq/24 hours
Uric acid levels: 250 to 750 mg/24 hours

HEPATITIS TESTING

H epatitis is a viral inflammation of the liver. Measurements of liver function are not really adequate to screen blood for the presence of a virus that causes serum hepatitis. Very few carriers of the virus are actually jaundiced. Therefore, carriers of the virus may show a mild derangement of more sensitive parameters like serum transaminases. Most specific are tests that detect the virus itself.

Hepatitis A is a liver infection caused by the hepatitis A virus and is vaccine preventable. Hepatitis A is very contagious and found in the stools and blood. Accidental ingestion of the virus even in microscopic amounts due to close contact with an infected person or through eating contaminated food can cause the infection. The symptoms are jaundice, nausea, fatigue and vomiting. The best prevention of a hepatitis A infection is getting a vaccination. The diagnosis of an acute hepatitis A virus (HAV) infection should show the presence of immunoglobulin M (IgM) as the standard.

The viral hepatitis B infection is caused by the hepatitis B virus. The spread of this infection occurs through blood, semen, saliva, and other body fluids. The transmission can occur by the sexual route, sharing needles and syringes, vertical transmission from the mother to the baby during delivery, and breastfeeding. The symptoms of hepatitis B include nausea, vomiting, fatigue and jaundice. Many carriers can remain asymptomatic.

Hepatitis B can be a short-term infection for some while for others it can turn into a chronic issue that can lead to other health conditions like cirrhosis and liver cancer. The presence of IgM for hepatitis B core antigen (HBcAg) in serum is required to confirm an acute hepatitis B virus (HBV) infection. In acute infection hepatitis B, surface antigen (HBsAg) is present and a hepatitis B core antibody test is done to see if the patient has ever been infected. The hepatitis B surface antibody suggests that the virus has been cleared after infection. The hepatitis B antigen may also be seen in patients who are chronic carriers. Patients with clinical symptoms of acute hepatitis along with the detection of virus strongly suggest acute HBV infection. It could also be chronic

HBV with acute superinfection by another hepatitis virus. A chronic hepatitis infection is the presence of HBsAg in the serum for 6 months or longer. The best mode of preventing this infection is by vaccination.

Hepatitis C is a viral infection of the liver caused by the hepatitis C virus. It usually gets transmitted through contact with the blood of an infected person. The most common route is sharing needles and other equipment used to inject drugs. Most often hepatitis C is a long-term infection which can lead to advanced liver disease and hepatic cancer. Patients with hepatitis C are usually asymptomatic, but when they present with symptoms, they are usually in advanced liver disease.

The best mode to avoid this infection is to avoid contact with blood-contaminating objects and recreational drugs. Serologic assays are done to detect antibody to HCV (anti-HCV), or molecular tests are done for the presence of viral particles to confirm hepatitis C virus (HCV) infection. Anti-HCV antibodies can be detected within 4-10 weeks of infection by third generation tests which are more sensitive and specific. A rapid test made up of antibody strips is also available. The polymerase chain reaction (PCR) assay done for HCV infection is the most specific test for presence of viral particles and is helpful in diagnosing acute HCV infection before antibodies have developed.

Hepatitis D is an infection in the liver caused by the hepatitis D virus, also called delta virus. This infection is usually seen in patients along with hepatitis B, where it is called a "co-infection". It can occur later in a patient already infected with hepatitis B, which is called "superinfection". Hepatitis D can be a short-term or a long-term infection that causes serious liver damage and even death. There isn't a vaccine that can block this infection, but vaccination against hepatitis B can offer protection against hepatitis D as well. Patients with a suspected hepatitis D infection are not routinely tested for the presence of IgM antibodies to hepatitis D virus (HDV). These infections can occur as superinfections with other hepatitis viruses.

Hepatitis E is an infection produced by the hepatitis E virus. The infection is spread by the stool of an infected person. In most developing countries, drinking contaminated water with the stool of an infected person causes the infection. In developed countries, hepatitis E occurs due to ingestion of undercooked or raw pork, shellfish, and wild boar meat. Patients are usually asymptomatic, but immunocompromised patients present with symptoms.

Imaging studies are not indicated to make the diagnosis of hepatitis. Imaging studies like ultrasonography or computed tomography [CT]) are done to rule out other differential diagnoses like biliary obstruction, gallbladder disease, or liver abscess.

Serological tests are highly specific for hepatitis virus markers. These tests include enzyme-linked immunosorbent assay (ELISA), radioimmunoassay, and microparticle enzyme immunoassay. The accuracy and precision of this technique and the fact that it is relatively easy to perform means that it has replaced most other techniques for identifying the presence of hepatitis virus in the serum.

NURSING IMPLICATIONS
If radionuclides are injected within 1 week before the blood test is performed, it may cause falsely elevated results in the radioimmunoassay.

Hepatitis A: the presence of immunoglobulin M (IgM) antibody to hepatitis A and presence of total antibody (IgG and IgM) may suggest an ongoing hepatitis A infection.

Hepatitis B: presence of Hep B core antigen (HBcAg), envelope antigen (HBeAg), and surface antigen (HBsAg), or their corresponding antibodies.

Hepatitis C: Diagnosed by the presence of antibodies to hep C virus.

Hepatitis D: Early detection of Hep D antigen (HDAg) in the course of infection and presence of Hepatitis D virus antibody in later stages of the disease.

Hepatitis E: Serological tests for hepatitis E virus include detection of specific IgM and IgG antibodies to hepatitis E.

THERAPEUTIC DRUG LEVELS

The monitoring of therapeutic levels of medications becomes paramount when the patient is on medications with a very narrow therapeutic range, where even a slight imbalance could be detrimental and critical. Therapeutic drug monitoring involves the measurement of the concentration of certain drugs in the patient's serum to optimize individual drug dosages.

Blood samples are drawn to monitor for peak and trough levels and to see if the blood serum levels of a spcific drug are within the therapeutic range and not at a toxic or subtherapeutic level. The highest drug concentration in the blood serum is represented by the peak level, while the trough level represents the lowest concentration.

NORMAL RANGES
- Phenobarbital (Luminal): 10 to 30 mcg/mL
- Phenytoin (Dilantin): 10 to 20 mcg/mL
- Lithium: 0.5 to 1.2 mEq/L
- Salicylate:100 to 250 mcg/mL
- Theophylline: 10 to 20 mcg/dL
- Tobramycin (Tobrex): 5 – 10 mcg/mL (peak); 0.5 – 2.0 mcg/mL (trough)
- Valproic acid (Depakene): 50 – 100 mcg/mL
- Magnesium sulfate: 4 to 7 mg/dL
- Vancomycin (Vancocin): 20 – 40 mcg/mL (peak); 5 – 15 mcg/mL (trough)Acetaminophen (Tylenol): 10 to 20 mcg/mL
- Carbamazepine (Tegretol): 5 to 12 mcg/mL
- Digoxin (Lanoxin): 0.5 to 2 ng/mL
- Gentamicin (Garamycin): 5 – 10 mcg/mL (peak); <2.0 mcg/mL (trough)

EASY MEMORIZATION TRICKS

Complete Blood Count

- **RBC, Hemoglobin, Hematocrit, ESR, Serum Ferritin and RBC indices (MCV, MCH, MCHC)**

The RBC count is about 5 million cells, that is, RBCs (4-6 million)

RBCs multiplied by 3 get the value of normal Hemoglobin (Hb), which is 15 g/dL or RBCs should be multiplied by 25 to get the SI units, which is 125 mmol/L

Hemoglobin value in men is 14-18 g/dL and for women 12-16 g/dL

The rule of thumb is that hematocrit is three times hemoglobin

For hematocrit value, the Hb is multiplied by 3, which is 45%

Hematocrit for men is 42-52% and for women 37–47%

The Early Settling Rate for marriage is within 30 years. (ESR 0-30mm)

RBC indices:

RBC indices are derived from three formulas having RBC two times, Hb two times and Hct two times in the formulas

MCV=Hct/RBC x 10; MCH= Hb/RBC x 10; MCHC= Hb/Hct x 100

Remember:

If it has 3 letters in the name it gets RBC AS DENOMINATOR

If it has H in the name it gets Hb AS NUMERATOR

The remaining two spots get HEMATOCRIT

MCV and MCH have x10; MCHC has x 100 (more letters gets a 100)

"A Strong Ferry is made up of about 60-160 iron rods."

Serum Iron/ Serum Ferritin: average value is 60-160

White Blood Count and differential count

WBC: 4000 -11000 cells

She saved 4000 - 10000 pounds and put it in the <u>W</u>orld <u>B</u>anking <u>C</u>onsortium

The differential count percentages in WBC can vary, but average percentages can be memorized.

"No Lesson is More Easy than Biology."

60, 30, 6, 3, 1

Neutrophils: 60% (range: 55-70% or 1,800 to 7,800 cells/mm³)

Lymphocytes 30% (range: 20-40% or 1,000 to 4,800 cells/mm³)

Monocytes 6% (range: 2-8% or 0.0 to 800 cells/mm³)

Eosinophils 3% (range: 1-4% or 0.0 to 450 cells/mm³)

Basophils 1% (range: 0-2% 0.0 to 200 cells/mm³)

Coagulation Studies

<u>A</u> <u>P</u>erfect <u>T</u>eaching <u>T</u>utor: <u>30- 40 </u>years (aPTT 30-40 Seconds)
<u>P</u>re-<u>t</u>een : 10-15 years   (PT 10-15 seconds)
<u>I</u>NR : 1

<u>B</u>efore <u>t</u>hree minutes: 1-3 (BT 1-3 minutes)

Mnemonic: **"Please <u>D</u>on't <u>D</u>ie before visiting 500 places in life"**

D-Dimer < 500

"Pat learned to eat in a <u>plate</u> when he was <u>1.5 - 4</u> years of age "

Platelets: 1.5 - 4 lakhs

Serum Electrolytes

Maggie and Phoebe are 1.6- 2.6 years old (magnesium and phosphorus)

They ate 3.5 - 5 bananas (potassium)

They drank 8.5- 10.5 oz of milk (calcium)

Then they took a 135 -145 minute nap after swimming in the ocean (sodium)

But they can only swim in the swimming pool at a temperature of 95 - 105 (chloride)

Renal studies

BUN - think of the price of a bun. It costs about $5 but no more than $20 (5-20)

Creatinine - an ugly creature on a scale of one to ten measures about 0.5 to 1.5 (0.5-1.5)

Glucose studies

Fasting glucose - think sweet candies. I eat 70-110 candies when I am hungry.

<u>Glucose Tolerance Test</u>

Baseline Glucose – "A child between 7-11 years plays with glue." Hence the values are 70-110

Baseline: 70-110

Remember that 120 comes 2 times diagonally, and the other numbers are 70 and 170

1 hour: 120 - 170

2 hours: 70 -120

HbA1c - think of numbers 3,4,5,6 - the average of glucose levels over 3 months and should be between 4-6

Arterial blood gas

Remember: pH 7.35 - 7.45
PaCO2 35- 45 (same as numbers after decimal points)

Bicarb- HCO3 22- 26 (between the ages of 22-26 we can buy cars)

Pao2 80- 100 (a person's old age is between 80-100 years)

SaO2 > 95 (you are super old when you cross 95 years of age)

Liver function tests

Remember that AST and ALT have the same ranges.

ALT - Liver specific in the range of 10-40

AST- System specific (not liver specific) in the range of 10-40

Remember that ALP and lipase have the same ranges.

ALP - Liver specific disease in the range of 10- 140

Lipase- Pancreatitis specific in the range of 10-140

Amylase - 40-140 (the same second value as the ALP and lipase)

Bilirubin - 0.1-1.0 (reverse the numbers in the values)

Lipoprotein profile and cardiac enzymes

Triglycerides: <200 (want low as bad fats in the bloodstream)

LDL - < 130 mg/dl (want LOW or it will lower you to the ground)

HDL - >30 mg/dl (want HIGH for patient to feel in high spirit)

Cardiac enzymes

Mnemonic: "The Assistant Commissioner of Police TICKs me off Totally and My Blood boils when I see him "

Acute Cardiac Profile (ACP)

The first enzyme to rise is troponin T >0.4 (specific in myocardial infarction)

followed by troponin I >0.1 (specific in myocardial infarction)

and then creatinine kinase CK-MB >50 (more specific than the CK-Total)

Creatinine kinase CK -Total >150 (more specific in muscle injury)

Myoglobin - 5-70 (more specific in muscle injury)

BNP <100

HIV and AIDS testing

Patients with HIV and AIDS - **LACK IMMU**nity

Lymphoid cells are most commonly affected

Autoimmunity is a feature of a HIV

CD4+ t cell molecule is downregulated

Killing of CD4+ T cells by cytotoxic T lymphocytes

Inability of T cells to proliferate when there is decrease in the T Helper cells

Merging of the CD4 cells by the virus (fusion)

Macrophage defects are seen in HIV

Unresponsiveness to the HIV infected CD8 cells after the early stages

Thyroid studies

Triiodothyronine (T3), Thyroxine (T4) and Thyroid Stimulating Hormone(TSH) - the test values decrease in descending order from T3 having the highest numbers to TSH having the lowest numbers.

T3 - 75-200 ng/dl

T4 - 4.5- 11.5 ug/dl

TSH - 0.3 - 5.0 U/dl

Urine Analysis

The most common crystals in urine are:

Calcium oxalate – the most common crystals that are envelope shaped (the most common shape we see because we send and receive email all the time)

URic acid - is rhomboid in shape

Cystine crystals - cys sounds like six and is hexagonal in shape

Struvite crystals - most fatal and are coffin shaped (a coffin is fatal)

Hepatitis

Hepatitis A, B, C, D and E

- The Hepatitis A and E which have a **vowel** come from the **bowel**

 Route of transmission: fecal and oral

- Hepatitis **B** comes from **Body fluids** that is blood, semen and saliva

- Hepatitis **C** comes from **Circulation** and by transfusion of blood

- Hepatitis **D** comes with **D**ouble infection (superinfection) from HBV.

Hepatitis A and B **have** vaccines

Hepatitis C, D and E **DO NOT** have vaccines

NOTES

_____

_____

_____

_____

_____

_____

_____

A SIMPLE STORY TO REMEMBER IMPORTANT LABORATORY VALUES

T his is a story of a rock band called, "Heavy Momentum", that conducted tours and concerts across the country. The band consisted of one man (heme) and 4 women (oxygen).

Hemoglobin is made up of 1 heme and 4 oxygen. Therefore,

Hemoglobin:

Men - 14-18 g/dl (the numbers are 1 and 4)

Women - 12- 16 g/dl (minus 2 from men's values)

There are forums that keep a check of these band performances, called "critiques" because they criticize their work. The critiques forum has about 42 to 52 men and 37 to 47 women.

Hematocrit:

Men 42-52%

Women 37-47%

The payment of the band singers is decided by a Really Backward Council known for pay disparity based on gender. Hence the men get paid 4.7- 6.1 million dollars and the women get paid 4.2- 5.4 million dollars, which is less than their male counterparts.

RBC:

Men 4.7 - 6.1 million cells / cumm

Women 4.2 - 5.4 million cells / cumm

At the same time, there is a council fighting for women's rights called the Women Backing Council that will penalize any forum creating pay disparity based on gender, with a fine of 4000 - 11000 dollars.

WBC 4000 - 11000 cells / cumm

The Heavy Momentum players have some older players called, cholesterol, who are on the higher side of age, who are really good singers, and these men are between 40 to 50 years; the women are between 50 to 60 years of age.

They also have a few very laidback members who are really bad singers aged between 60-180 years

HDL (good cholesterol) Men: 40 - 50 and Women: 50 - 60

LDL (bad cholesterol) 60 -180

The audience includes Aunt Thea, who has come with her family of 10 to 20 people. They all want to eat a hamburger Bun, which costs about 5 dollars to 20 dollars, depending upon the filling inside. These buns are served on plates arranged in stacks of 150000 to 450000 lakhs for the entire audience.

Theophylline 10 - 20 mcg

BUN (blood urea nitrogen) 5-20

Platelets - 150000 - 450000 lakhs

The audience can also avail itself of a free dessert if it has a glucose level within the normal range of 70 - 110 mg/dl. And they get a chance to win a pass to meet and greet the band members backstage if they have exhibited fair and good behavior in other concerts over three months. If they have misbehaved more than 6.5 times in the last three months, they automatically get disqualified from winning the pass.

Normal glucose: 70 - 110 mg/dl

HbA1c Good control 5.7 - 6.5 % over three months

Diabetes >6.5%

A great singer who is very experienced called Patrick charges about 3.5 - 5 million dollars for each concert hosted and sponsored by lithium. Patrick is the brand ambassador for lithium, and he carries lithium bottles with him everywhere and consumes 0.6 to 1.2 liters of it. Also, there is another new singer on the block, Albert, who is extremely good but also charges the same rate of 3.5 - 5 million dollars. Therefore, this band could not afford him and they let him go.

Potassium (K+) 3.5 - 5

Albumin 3.5 - 5

Lithium 0.6 - 1.2

Patrick was accused of doing drugs and, therefore, he had to undergo a battery of tests that included a urine analysis. His urinalysis and blood protein showed the following results which were normal.

ALB 0-8mg/dl

pH 4.6 - 8.0

WBC 0-4

Glucose Negative

And his blood test showed:

 Protein 6.4 - 8.3g/dl.

Patrick and another standby band member, Socrates, are at loggerheads and share a bitter relationship because Patrick went out with Amy, who is Socrates' wife, at least 35-65 times. Also when Patrick is playing in the band, Socrates rests and vice versa because of their complicated love story. They do not play in the band at the same time.

Potassium 3.5 - 5 mEq/dl

Sodium 135 -145 mEq/dl

Ammonia 35-65 mcg/dl

Socrates and Amy have a daughter, Maggie, who is 1.6 -2.6 years old (magnesium). She came to the concert and was hungry. She had 8.5 - 10.5 oz of milk (calcium). After the concert, her parents took her to the swimming pool (chloride) where she swam for 90 - 105 minutes.

Magnesium 1.6 -2.6

Calcium 8.5 - 10.5

Chloride 90 - 105

In the meantime, after the exertion of the concert, Patrick complained of tightness in his chest and was suddenly gasping for breath. He was rushed to the emergency room and a series of tests were ordered. His oxygen levels were more than 95%, but the Trop I test was also more than 0.4. He was also tested for HIV because of his drug addiction. The test turned out positive but his Cd4+ cell count was between 500 – 1000, which was normal. He was informed by the doctors that he had had a heart attack and he should slow down. He then decided to resign from the band due to his health conditions.

Spo2 >95%

Trop I > 0.4 (indicates myocardial infarction)

HIV cd4 cell count normal range: 500 -1000

The band found a new member, Phoenix, to replace Patrick who was extremely talented and also charges only 1.8 to 2.6 million dollars per concert - less than Patrick charged. It was a win-win situation for both Phoenix and the band.

Phosphorus 1.8 - 2.6 mEq/dl

CONCLUSION

The ultimate goal for registered nurses and students is to have accurate and simple information and to make learning lab values easy for nursing students and working nurses. This book is written as a guide to provide a valuable aid throughout one's nursing career and especially to those taking their exams. Lab values form an important part of the NCLEX exams, and it is essential for nursing students to remember normal ranges and critical values to do well. This book keeps learning simple and helps students focus on the most important aspects of laboratory tests ordered in the hospital.

Nursing lab values primarily consist of numbers that can be very dry and difficult to remember. The last two chapters, "Easy Memorization Tricks" and "The Story" aimed to make absorbing these values fun and easy. When mnemonics and stories are silly, it makes for an easy read for students and helps them retain the material longer. These tricks come at the end of the book so that glancing through these values in a concise manner becomes manageable when exams approach.

NOTES

_____

_____

_____

_____

_____

_____

_____

_____

_____

_____

_____

CPSIA information can be obtained
at www.ICGtesting.com
Printed in the USA
LVHW050756120221
679113LV00016B/552